Mnemonics for Radiologists and Professional Exam Preparation

A systematic approach

PHILIP YOONG

Clinical Fellow in Musculoskeletal Radiology
Nuffield Orthopaedic Centre, Oxford

WILLIAM BUGG

Radiology Registrar
Norfolk and Norwich University Hospital

and

CATHERINE A JOHNSON

Senior Fellow in Radiology
Royal Marsden Hospital, London

Foreword by
DR ANDONI TOMS
Consultant Radiologist
Norfolk and Norwich University Hospital

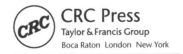

CRC Press
Taylor & Francis Group
Boca Raton London New York

CRC Press is an imprint of the
Taylor & Francis Group, an **informa** business

CRC Press
Taylor & Francis Group
6000 Broken Sound Parkway NW, Suite 300
Boca Raton, FL 33487-2742

Printed on acid-free paper
Version Date: 20150928

International Standard Book Number-13: 978-1-908911-95-7 (Paperback)

Visit the Taylor & Francis Web site at
http://www.taylorandfrancis.com

and the CRC Press Web site at
http://www.crcpress.com

Contents

Foreword

The art of mnemonics has been at the root of scholarship for millennia. In ancient Greece to be an authority with the power to speak in public required you to possess Mnemosyne, the Titaness daughter of Gaia and Uranus, the personification of memory. After death the new arrivals in Hades would be given a choice: to drink from the river Lethe to forget their past lives or to drink from the river Mnemosyne to remember. Embarking on the Fellowship examination is just the same.

Scholars from the Greek Sophists to Roger Bacon and Giordano Bruno spent much of their lives perfecting mnemonic systems in a world where data storage, in the form of parchment and paper, were expensive and where the Lamarckian inheritance of culture and education was an oral tradition. In today's world where all information is instantly available through a touch-sensitive screen, rote learning can at first seem an archaic and all too prosaic task but we do still need mnemonics.

Mnemonics, and the related system of loci, are more effective for learning new vocabularies than other contextual and free learning methods.[1] For the trainee the vocabulary of radiology is certainly new. So when faced with the daunting task of learning seemingly unintelligible lists for exams this is the technique of choice. At first glance the short-term aim of exam success may seem a transient achievement but the series of rote learned lists provides the new radiologist with a framework for his knowledge on the subject. A framework that may at first be learned but not fully understood; a framework that allows each piece of knowledge to be juxtaposed and compared with its neighbour; a framework that will be broken, rebuilt and remodelled by personal experience; one that will be the start of a lifelong expertise.

This book is a recipe book of mnemonics. Like all the best recipe books each has been tried and tested as the authors devised them to get them through their FRCR examinations. And like all recipes some you will like as they are, and others you will adapt and flavour to your own taste. They will all be memorable.

Dr Andoni Toms
Consultant Radiologist
Norfolk and Norwich University Hospital
June 2013

Reference

1 Levin JR, Nordwall MB. Mnemonic vocabulary instruction: additional effectiveness evidence. *Contemporary Educational Psychology.* 1992; **17**(2): 156–74.

Preface

Revising for the final FRCR examination is a challenging task. You must balance your revision time between image interpretation practice, learning facts and refining presentation skills. While it is better to gain an understanding of the underlying mechanisms that result in a radiological abnormality, it is an unavoidable truth that some things just have to be rote learned. This involves long lists of differential diagnoses, which include both frequently seen and exceptionally rare conditions. Some of these rarer topics are more frequently encountered in the exam than in normal day-to-day radiology practice.

It can be difficult to memorise the numerous conditions associated with a certain radiological appearance. We believe mnemonics can be of assistance. A mnemonic is a tool used to aid information retention. The word originates from Ancient Greek and the name for the goddess of memory, Mnemosyne. Mnemonics in medical practice typically use word-based cues to enhance memory, reduce cognitive load and aid learning. In this book, each mnemonic is either an acronym (an abbreviation, pronounced as a word, formed from the first letters of several particular pieces of information) or an acrostic (a sentence in which the first letter of each word refers to a piece of information beginning with the same letter). Some are well known to radiology and others are the product of our sleep-deprived imagination. We found mnemonics very useful not only in aiding our rote learning but also in organising our revision.

Each case shown in this book is presented in the same way. First, a film is presented with a radiological finding for which there is a set of differential diagnoses. This is followed by a mnemonic, listing the most relevant diagnoses with the exam in mind. For each stem of each mnemonic, the main radiological findings and useful distinguishing features are listed. A model answer is given for each case, written as you might present it in the viva examination. A short discussion of the main diagnoses follows, with some practical advice and some tips and tricks that may make your life easier.

This book does not aim to list every possible differential diagnosis associated with each particular radiological finding presented. There are very good, much larger books that do this already. We recommend that you use these books in combination with our own when preparing for the exam. We aim to demonstrate a mechanism for organising your thoughts, focusing your revision on the more important diagnoses and providing some clarity when confronted with the mountain of information that you will be expected to retain and recall during your all-important viva examination and throughout your career.

Good luck!

Philip Yoong
William Bugg
Catherine A Johnson
June 2013

About the authors

Philip Yoong is a clinical fellow in musculoskeletal radiology at the Nuffield Orthopaedic Centre, Oxford. He graduated from University College London in 2002 and completed basic surgical training before joining the Norwich radiology training scheme in 2008.

William Bugg is a final year radiology registrar at the Norfolk and Norwich University Hospital. He graduated from Imperial College London in 2002 and completed basic surgical training before joining the Norwich radiology training scheme in 2008. His subspecialty areas of interest are gastrointestinal and musculoskeletal radiology.

Catherine A Johnson is a senior fellow in radiology at the Royal Marsden Hospital, London. She graduated from Imperial College London in 2002. After completing her basic surgical training, she trained as a radiologist in East Anglia and London. She completed her radiology training in 2013. Her subspecialty areas of interest are oncology, genitourinary, and head and neck radiology.

Acknowledgement

The authors would like to thank Mr Roger Bugg for his help with the manuscript.

Dedication

To Richard Joseph Yoong, the boy who never slept. PY and CAJ

To Megan, Charlotte and my family, with love. WB

Abbreviations

ABC	aneurysmal bone cyst
ADC	apparent diffusion coefficient
AP	antero-posterior
ARDS	acute respiratory distress syndrome
AVN	avascular necrosis
AXR	abdominal X-ray (abdominal radiograph)
CEP	chronic eosinophilic pneumonia
CNS	central nervous system
COP	cryptogenic organising pneumonia
CP	cerebellopontine
CSF	cerebrospinal fluid
CT	computed tomography
CXR	chest X-ray (chest radiograph)
DWI	diffusion-weighted imaging
EAA	extrinsic allergic alveolitis
ERCP	endoscopic retrograde cholangiopancreatography
ESR	erythrocyte sedimentation rate
fatsat	fat saturation
FLAIR	fluid-attenuated inversion recovery
FNH	focal nodular hyperplasia
FRCR	Fellow of the Royal College of Radiologists
GBM	glioblastoma multiforme
GCT	giant cell tumour
GGO	ground-glass opacification
HCC	hepatocellular carcinoma
HOA	hypertrophic osteoarthropathy
HRCT	high resolution computed tomography
IAM	internal acoustic meatus
IV	intravenous
IVC	inferior vena cava
IVU	intravenous urography
LAM	lymphangioleiomyomatosis

MDT	multidisciplinary team
MIBG	metaiodobenzylguanidine
MR	magnetic resonance
MRI	magnetic resonance imaging
NF-1	neurofibromatosis type 1
NF-2	neurofibromatosis type 2
NSIP	non-specific interstitial pneumonia
PAH	pulmonary artery hypertension
PCP	pneumocystis pneumonia
PE	pulmonary effusion
PIP	proximal interphalangeal
P-LCH	pulmonary Langerhans' cell histiocytosis
PMF	progressive massive fibrosis
PTH	parathyroid hormone
PUJ	pelviureteric junction
RA	rheumatoid arthritis
RPN	renal papillary necrosis
STIR	short tau inversion recovery
TB	tuberculosis
TS	tuberous sclerosis
UC	ulcerative colitis
VZV	*Varicella zoster virus*

Section 1

Cardiorespiratory

1.
Upper lobe fibrosis

"STREP ABC"

	Condition	Associated features
S	Sarcoidosis	"Egg-shell" calcification of lymph nodes Hilar/mediastinal adenopathy Background lung nodularity
T	Tuberculosis (TB; secondary)	Cavitating lung lesions
R	Radiation	Well-defined non-anatomical border with normal lung Evidence of previous surgery (mastectomy, surgical clips)
E	Extrinsic allergic alveolitis (EAA)	
P	Pneumoconiosis Progressive massive fibrosis (PMF)	Conglomerate upper lobe masses "Egg-shell" calcification of lymph nodes Background lung nodularity
A	Ankylosing spondylitis	Ankylosis of cervical spine
C	Cystic fibrosis	Young patient Portacath

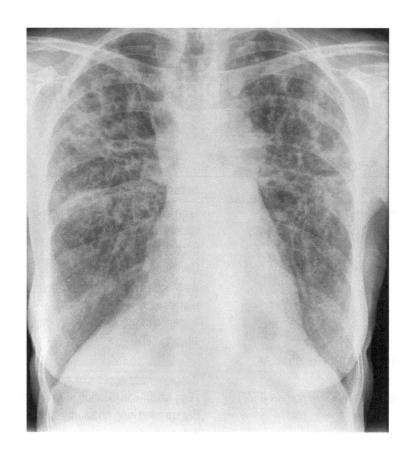

Diagnosis: Stage IV sarcoidosis

Definition: Fibrosis of the upper lobes with associated volume loss and architectural distortion, typically bilateral

---

MODEL ANSWER

This is a frontal chest radiograph of an adult female patient. There is extensive reticular shadowing and architectural distortion in both upper lobes. There is upper lobe volume loss resulting in hilar elevation. The lower zones are relatively spared. The aortopulmonary window and the right paratracheal region are bulky, in keeping with mediastinal lymphadenopathy. There is no lymph node calcification. The features are of bilateral upper lobe fibrosis.

The most likely diagnosis is advanced sarcoidosis given the presence of mediastinal lymphadenopathy. However, the differential diagnoses include tuberculosis and progressive massive fibrosis.

To take this further, I would review the patient's clinical history and any previous imaging to assess for disease progression. The patient should be referred to the chest clinic. An HRCT [high resolution computed tomography] scan would be useful to provide a more detailed assessment of the lung parenchyma and mediastinum.

Discussion

There are two different themes to a film showing bilateral upper lobe fibrosis. One will be an "Aunt Minnie", with a giveaway additional feature such as that described (e.g. a portacath – an implanted venous access device). The other will require a good description of the findings, the provision of a sensible list of differential diagnoses (such as sarcoidosis, TB and pneumoconiosis) and a good management plan.

Pneumoconiosis is due to the accumulation of inhaled dust particles in the lung. Silicosis and coal worker's pneumoconiosis are the two best-known forms. Pneumoconiosis may either be simple (resulting in multiple small lung nodules) or complicated (resulting in PMF, which is seen bilaterally in the upper lobes).

It is difficult to distinguish between sarcoidosis, TB and pneumoconiosis on a single chest radiograph. However, some findings are more common in one or more of these conditions than in others.

- Mediastinal lymphadenopathy is more common in sarcoidosis than secondary (reactivation) TB.
- Cavitating lung lesions are more frequently a feature of reactivation TB.
- Conglomerate perihilar upper lobe masses larger than 1 cm are more often seen in PMF.
- Peripheral "egg-shell" calcification of hilar lymph nodes is most commonly seen in silicosis but is also seen in coal worker's pneumoconiosis and sarcoidosis.
- Background nodularity of the lung parenchyma can be seen in any of these conditions.

Pearls

- Is the case an "Aunt Minnie"? Look at the lower cervical spine. Is there an unusual non-anatomical pattern of fibrosis? Is there a portacath in a young patient?
- On a radiograph showing bilateral upper lobe fibrosis without any specific distinguishing features, sarcoidosis, TB and complicated pneumoconiosis/PMF are the three most sensible possible diagnoses.
- Comment on the presence or absence of hilar/mediastinal lymphadenopathy, calcified lymph nodes and conglomerate upper lobe opacities.
- A history of foreign travel, previous radiotherapy, industrial exposure to dust or exposure to an allergen (birds etc.) may lead you to the specific diagnosis. You may have to ask for this information after listing your differential diagnoses.
- Suggest comparison with previous imaging to assess for disease progression.
- Suggest referral to the respiratory physicians, if the patient is not already known to them.
- Further imaging with HRCT can help to distinguish between the possible differential diagnoses.

2.
Diffuse cystic interstitial lung disease without loss of lung volume

"LENT" or "Do not give up lung volumes for LENT"

	Condition	Associated features
L	Lymphangioleiomyomatosis (LAM)	Females of childbearing age only Pneumothorax Pleural effusion
E	Eosinophilic granuloma (pulmonary Langerhans' cell histiocytosis [P-LCH])	Commonly affects young adult males Nodules Pneumothorax
N	Neurofibromatosis type 1 (NF-1)	Dysplastic "ribbon" or eroded ribs Neurofibromas in the posterior mediastinum and subcutaneous tissues
T	Tuberous sclerosis (TS)	Pulmonary features identical to LAM

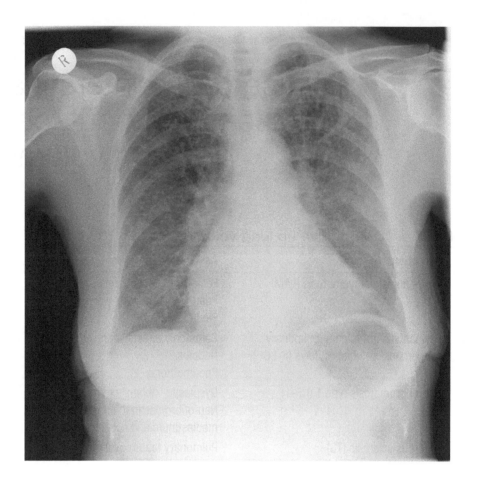

Diagnosis: P-LCH

MODEL ANSWER

This is a frontal chest radiograph of an adult female patient. There is diffuse reticulonodular shadowing throughout both lungs, without obvious zonal pre-dominance. There is no associated loss of lung volume. There is no blunting of the costophrenic angles to suggest a pleural effusion. No pneumothorax. The cardiomediastinal contour is unremarkable. No significant bony or subcutaneous soft tissue abnormality is demonstrated.

In summary, the findings are of diffuse interstitial lung disease with preserved lung volumes. As this is an adult female patient, lymphangioleiomyomatosis and P-LCH are the most likely diagnoses. Neurofibromatosis and tuberous sclerosis are also possible, but less likely causes.

I would like to know the patient's age, if there is a smoking history and to compare this film with any previous radiographs to assess for progression. I would refer the patient to the chest clinic and arrange for an HRCT for further assessment of the lung parenchyma.

Discussion

If you are presented with a chest radiograph (CXR) with features of interstitial lung disease in the exam, your pattern recognition skills are being tested. The key is to recognise the predominant pattern and distribution of the interstitial changes and to comment on the lung volumes (reduced, normal or increased). On the CXR, interstitial lung disease may present with a linear, reticular (mesh- or net-like), nodular or reticulonodular pattern. Recognising these features will help you to select the correct differential list and then to refine this to a shorter set of possible diagnoses. Further assessment of the film for associated secondary features may then bring you to the most likely diagnosis.

The overlapping walls of the multiple cysts seen in these conditions generate the reticular pattern demonstrated on the CXR. On the CXR shown, there are both linear and rounded solid densities, in keeping with a reticulonodular pattern. This distinction is very important, as an exclusively nodular pattern would alter the differential diagnoses to conditions such as sarcoidosis, TB, metastases and pneumoconioses.

Be careful – if you ask for an HRCT in the further management section of your answer (or even if you do not), you may be shown one. You will look a little silly if you then cannot read it! The key to the HRCT will probably be to see if you can distinguish between LAM and P-LCH.

P-LCH is characterised by centrilobular nodules, which cavitate into cysts that are often bizarrely shaped and of varying size and wall thickness. The distribution favours the mid and upper lobes, sparing the lung bases (this is not often apparent on chest radiography and much more easily demonstrated on computed tomography [CT]).

LAM is characterised by small (approximately 5 mm) cysts of uniform size with no zonal predominance. Nodules are not a feature.

Pattern recognition takes practice, through seeing many films. Being able to recite confidently your differential lists also takes practice. There is no short cut to success in these cases. However, once you have cracked it, it quickly becomes time well spent. If you are able to quickly and accurately assess these films and recite a focused list of differential diagnoses, you will inspire confidence in your examiners and do well. Scrabbling for the differential list has the opposite effect.

Pearls

- When confronted with a chest radiograph with abnormal lung parenchyma, first try to establish the primary pattern: lines, nodules or both? What are the lung volumes? If they are normal or increased, think "Do not give up lung volume for LENT!"
- Look for breast shadows in order to establish the sex of the patient. LAM only affects adult females of childbearing age. The examiner will not be impressed if you offer this in your differential list for a male patient.
- Smoking is strongly associated with P-LCH.

- Spontaneous recurrent pneumothoraces are associated with both LAM and P-LCH.
- A chylous pleural effusion is associated with LAM. Patients may also have chylous ascites.
- Interstitial lung disease is not a predominant feature in NF-1 (20% of cases) or TS (1% of cases). Nevertheless, it is worth looking for mediastinal masses, "ribbon" ribs, rib erosions and subcutaneous nodules (from neurofibromas) and commenting on the absence of these features.
- Make sure you can distinguish between P-LCH and LAM on HRCT. Look for nodules, cyst shape, cyst wall thickness, uniform cyst size and sparing of the lower zones.
- TS is a multisystem neurocutaneous disorder, involving the lungs, central nervous system (CNS), kidneys, heart and skeleton. It is therefore a diagnosis well suited to the long case section of the exam.
- Eosinophilic granuloma is synonymous with Langerhans' cell histiocytosis.

3.
Diffuse reticulonodular shadowing

"Sarcoidosis Does Like Producing Variable HRCT Findings"

	Condition	Associated features
S	Sarcoidosis	Reticulonodular opacities in the mid and upper zones Lobulated symmetrical hilar enlargement with right paratracheal stripe widening due to lymphadenopathy – Garland's triad Nodules along subpleural surfaces and bronchovascular bundles "Egg-shell" calcification of nodes Upper lobe fibrosis and traction bronchiectasis in end-stage disease
D	Drug reactions	Non-specific
L	Lymphangitis carcinomatosis	Evidence of malignancy, e.g. pulmonary nodules or masses, rib lesions, mastectomy, neck mass, mediastinal mass, surgical clips Pleural effusions Loss of lung volume Hilar and mediastinal lymphadenopathy
P	Pneumoconiosis	Hilar lymphadenopathy "Egg-shell" nodal calcification Conglomerate upper lobe masses (PMF) Upper lobe fibrosis
V	Viral pneumonia	Non-specific Nodal enlargement in children
H	Heart failure	Cardiomegaly Perihilar opacification Upper lobe venous distension Pleural effusions Kerley's lines
F	Fibrosis	Volume loss Lower zone predominance (collagen vascular disease, idiopathic, asbestosis) Pleural plaques (in asbestosis)

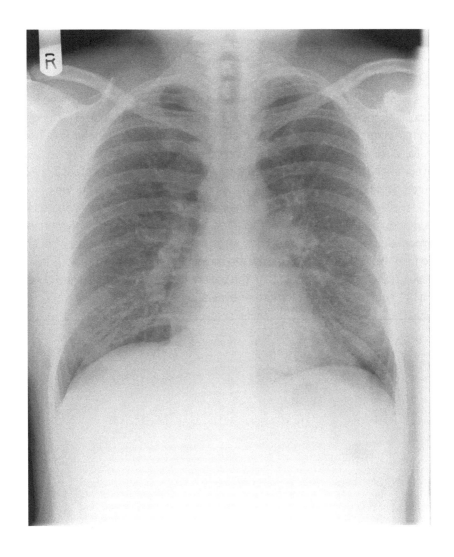

Diagnosis: Sarcoidosis

MODEL ANSWER

This is a frontal chest radiograph of an adult male patient. There is diffuse reticulonodular shadowing in both lungs without a zonal predominance. The lungs are of normal volume. Normal hilar and mediastinal contours. The heart is of normal size. No pleural or bony abnormality can be seen.

In summary, there is diffuse reticulonodular shadowing with no other significant features. This has a wide differential. If the patient were not acutely unwell, I would consider sarcoidosis and pneumoconioses such as silicosis and coal worker's pneumoconiosis. If the patient were acutely unwell, I would consider lymphangitis carcinomatosis, acute drug reactions, viral pneumonia and pulmonary oedema.

To take this further, I would review the clinical history and any previous imaging to assess for chronicity. I would refer the patient to a chest physician and consider an HRCT scan of the chest for further evaluation.

Discussion

Pathology in the lung interstitium is responsible for a reticulonodular pattern on CXR. The interstitium is the supporting tissue around the airways and contains lymphatics, connective tissue and pulmonary vasculature. On a normal CXR, the interstitium can be seen to mainly consist of pulmonary vessels. These are large and prominent at the hila and gradually reduce in size and prominence towards the periphery, becoming too small to see. Abnormality of the lung interstitium presents as increased lines (reticular), nodules (nodular), or lines and nodules (reticulonodular pattern). The abnormalities fall into two main categories: those caused by abnormal fluid in the interstitium (e.g. lymphangitis, pulmonary oedema) or inflammation of the interstitium (e.g. sarcoidosis, silicosis, idiopathic pulmonary fibrosis).

In contrast to interstitial disease, air space opacification is due to the filling of the gas-containing structures of the lung with fluid. There is usually a more homogeneous increased lung density with indistinct margins. Air bronchograms may be seen and are characteristic.

CXR is not specific or sensitive enough to diagnose subtle lung pathologies. It is not easy to spot or tell the difference between normal, hazy increased density, reticular, nodular or reticulonodular patterns. A useful technique is to focus on a small area of peripheral lung parenchyma and ask yourself, "Are there too many lines and/or nodules in this area? What is the predominant pattern?" Once you have established that, look for pertinent negatives that may help narrow the list of differential diagnoses. In most cases, HRCT is needed for further evaluation.

Pearls

- Always think of sarcoidosis when there is a diffuse reticulonodular pattern on CXR.
- When there is a large set of possible diagnoses, categorise them into those more likely if a patient is acutely unwell or well – this demonstrates your knowledge and reasoning.
- Look for the pertinent negatives such as lymphadenopathy, volume loss, cardiomegaly, pleural effusions or mastectomy.
- Further management with HRCT and referral to a chest physician is usually appropriate.
- Lymphangitis carcinomatosis is usually associated with adenocarcinoma, most commonly of the breast, lung, colon, stomach, pancreas and larynx.
- A mnemonic for the causes of lower lobe fibrosis is "CIA": Collagen vascular disease (e.g. rheumatoid, scleroderma), Idiopathic and Asbestosis.

4.
Multiple pulmonary nodules

"CAVITIES"

	Condition	Associated features
C	Cancer (metastatic or primary lung)	Features of malignancy Mastectomy, evidence of other surgery (e.g. surgical clips), lymphangitis, lymphadenopathy, bone lesions
A	Autoimmune (Wegener's granulomatosis, rheumatoid nodules)	Wegener's granulomatosis: • round lesions, which may show cavitation • no calcification Rheumatoid nodules: • peripheral and lower zone predominance • basal lung fibrosis • arthropathy
V	Vascular (infarcts, septic emboli)	Infarcts: • pulmonary artery enlargement • pulmonary embolus on CT scan Septic emboli: • cavitation • source of infection
I	Infection Inflammatory (granulomas, fungal, previous chickenpox pneumonia, multiple lung abscesses)	Associated consolidation Relevant clinical history
T	TB	Variable appearance Possible findings include consolidation, lymphadenopathy, upper lobe cavitation and pleural effusions
S	Sarcoidosis, silicosis and Langerhans' cell histiocytosis	Sarcoidosis: check for Garland's triad of lymphadenopathy Silicosis or other pneumoconioses: small nodules that may calcify Langerhans' cell histiocytosis: there may be cavitation of the larger nodules

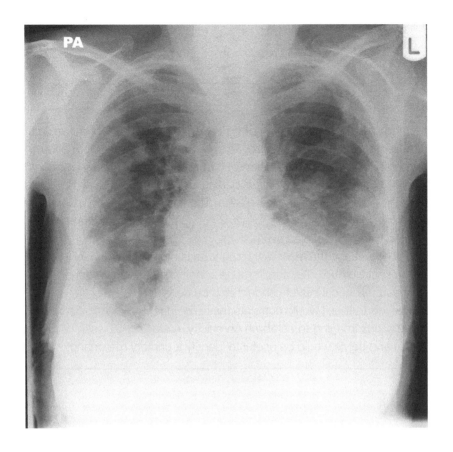

Diagnosis: Metastatic renal cell carcinoma

Definition: More than one pulmonary nodule (measuring between 2 and 30 mm, or larger than millet seeds)

MODEL ANSWER

This is a frontal chest radiograph of an adult female patient. There are multiple bilateral lung nodules of varying size. There is no cavitation or calcification. There are moderate bilateral pleural effusions. Normal cardiac and mediastinal contours. There is no soft tissue abnormality; in particular, no axillary surgical clips or asymmetry of the breast shadows can be seen. There are no aggressive bone lesions.

In summary, there are multiple, bilateral pulmonary nodules of non-uniform size associated with bilateral pleural effusions.

In an adult patient, the most likely diagnosis is multiple pulmonary metastases. However, septic emboli, TB, autoimmune conditions such as Wegener's granulomatosis and multifocal infarcts should also be considered.

To take this further, I would correlate these findings with the clinical history and review previous imaging to establish chronicity. A staging CT scan of the chest, abdomen and pelvis would be useful to identify a primary malignancy.

Discussion

This is one of the most common viva themes (probably in the top five). It may appear early in a viva exam, so it is important to give a polished performance. In the absence of any distinguishing features, it may not be possible to reach a diagnosis for a case of multiple lung nodules, so delivering a concise and organised list of differential diagnoses, as presented in the model answer, will help you to impress the examiner and move on to the next case as quickly as possible.

Metastatic disease is the most likely cause of multiple pulmonary nodules (larger than miliary nodules). Therefore, it is critical to scrutinise the film for evidence of malignancy. In particular, look for:

- mastectomy
- surgical clips in axilla, hilum or neck
- hilar and/or mediastinal lymphadenopathy
- absent humerus (implies previous osteosarcoma – a classic viva case)
- reticular shadowing (lymphangitis)
- lytic/sclerotic bone lesions (bony metastases).

Pearls

- The most likely cause of multiple pulmonary nodules of varying sizes is metastases.
- Look for evidence of malignancy (e.g. mastectomy, lymphangitis, surgical clips, lytic/sclerotic bone lesions).
- If the primary malignancy is not apparent, a CT scan of the chest, abdomen and pelvis is indicated to try and identify one.
- Also mention infection, autoimmune and vascular causes in your differential.
- This mnemonic can also apply to multiple cavitating lung nodules and solitary pulmonary nodules.

5.
Multiple small non-calcified (miliary) pulmonary nodules

"Test Match Special"

	Condition	Associated features
T	TB (miliary)	Superadded consolidation/cavitation Lymphadenopathy
M	Metastases	Lytic/sclerotic bony lesions Previous surgery (mastectomy, surgical clips in neck, axilla) Lymphangitis
S	Sarcoidosis Simple silicosis	Sarcoidosis: ● subpleural nodules – an HRCT feature ● bilateral hilar and right paratracheal lymphadenopathy ● "egg-shell" calcification of lymph nodes Simple silicosis: ● hilar and mediastinal lymphadenopathy ● "egg-shell" calcification of lymph nodes

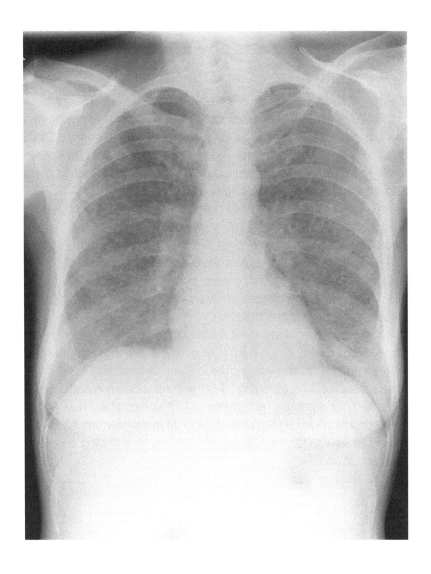

Diagnosis: Miliary TB

MODEL ANSWER

This is a frontal chest radiograph of an adult female patient. There are multiple, small, discrete, non-calcified nodules throughout both lungs. The pattern is uniform without a zonal predominance. The lung volumes are normal. There is no consolidation or cavitation. The cardiomediastinal contour is also normal. No bony abnormality is visible. There is no evidence of previous surgery, such as asymmetry of the breast shadows or metallic surgical clips.

In summary, there are multiple small pulmonary nodules throughout both lungs in a miliary pattern.

If the patient were unwell, the most likely diagnosis would be either miliary TB or metastatic disease. Primary tumours that may cause miliary metastases include thyroid, melanoma, breast, gastric, pancreatic, bronchus and prostate. If the patient were relatively well, I would also consider sarcoidosis and pneumoconioses such as uncomplicated silicosis.

Further management of this patient should include a review of their medical history for a previous malignancy. I would compare this film with any previous chest radiographs for signs of progression. The referring clinician should be informed of the findings. If appropriate, a staging CT of the chest, abdomen and pelvis may be useful to search for a primary malignancy or further metastatic disease. Sputum and blood cultures could be taken to assess for **Mycobacterium**. An HRCT could be obtained to assess for the features of sarcoidosis, including subpleural and bronchovascular nodules.

Discussion

Films showing multiple pulmonary nodules are common and can be divided into subcategories based on appearance: their size and the presence or absence of calcification and cavitation. This case shows multiple small non-calcified pulmonary nodules.

Traditionally, nodules of 1–4 mm in size are described as miliary, in reference to the size of millet seed. It may be more useful to call these "small pulmonary nodules" when they can be discerned on CXR.

Miliary TB is an uncommon manifestation of TB that occurs predominantly in older people and those who are immunocompromised, resulting from blood-borne dissemination of bacilli. It is seen in less than 10% of patients with TB and may be a sequela of both primary infection and secondary reactivation. Therefore, there are sometimes superadded features of both primary (mediastinal adenopathy, consolidation) and reactivation (upper lobe cavitation) TB. Unfortunately for the exam setting, these features are also often absent.

Sarcoidosis is a multisystem disorder, and an exam favourite. The majority of patients will have thoracic disease. The classical CXR feature is of bilateral hilar and right paratracheal lymphadenopathy. The lung nodules may have a mid and upper zone predominance. Assessment with HRCT will reveal subpleural nodules, such as on the fissures and bronchovascular bundles.

Uncomplicated/simple silicosis results from long-term (>20 years) exposure to free silica, commonly industrial or occupational. Radiological presentation is with multiple bilateral lung nodules less than 1 cm in diameter, with associated hilar and mediastinal lymphadenopathy. As the disease progresses to complicated silicosis, these small nodules coalesce to form larger nodules (>1 cm) that tend to migrate from the lung periphery towards the hila.

Pearls

- Establish that the pattern is of small, non-calcified, diffuse pulmonary nodules.
- Look for mediastinal lymphadenopathy, consolidation/cavitation and evidence of malignancy (bony lesions, mastectomy, lymphangitis, surgical clips).
- Miliary metastases are classically thyroid in origin.
- Miliary TB nodules do not calcify. Calcified pulmonary nodules have a different set of differential diagnoses such as healed *Varicella zoster virus* (VZV; chickenpox) pneumonia (*see* Case 6).
- This mnemonic also applies to random nodules on HRCT.

6.
Multiple calcified lung nodules

"SHAMPOO"

	Condition	Associated features
S	Silicosis	Silicosis – chronic simple: • well-defined small nodules • mid and upper zone predominance • "egg-shell" calcification of hilar and/or mediastinal nodes Silicosis – complicated: • irregular conglomerate lung masses (PMF) • initially peripheral mass, with migration towards the hilum
H	Histoplasmosis Hyperparathyroidism	Histoplasmosis (healed): • small, well-defined, acute nodules develop into multiple punctate calcifications • hilar and mediastinal lymphadenopathy • "popcorn" calcification of large mediastinal nodes • upper lobe fibrosis/cavitation (similar to TB) • punctate splenic calcifications (more visible on CT) Hyperparathyroidism: • rare • ill-defined, may be large lung lesions • lateral clavicle resorption • superior/inferior rib notching • osteopenia/osteosclerosis • soft tissue calcification
A	Alveolar microlithiasis	Tiny, sand-like, diffuse calcifications that can obscure normal lung markings Diffuse involvement of both lungs Calcium uptake demonstrated on bone scan Usually asymptomatic

	Condition	Associated features
M	Metastases Mitral stenosis	Metastases: • may be large, randomly distributed and of varying size • evidence of bony abnormality – lysis/sclerosis/absent limb, e.g. proximal humerus (osteosarcoma) • neck mass/surgery (thyroid carcinoma) Mitral stenosis: • small diffuse nodules • mid and lower zone predominance • cardiomegaly • double right heart border, splayed carina
P	Previous chickenpox (VZV) infection	Well-defined small nodules of similar size No zonal predominance No calcified lymph nodes

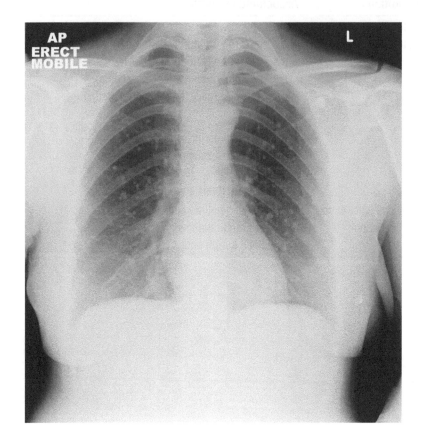

Diagnosis: Healed varicella (Chickenpox) pneumonia

MODEL ANSWER

This is a mobile AP [antero-posterior] erect chest radiograph of an adult female patient. There are multiple, small, well-defined, calcified lung nodules in both lungs. The lungs are normal volume. There is no consolidation or pulmonary mass. No hilar or mediastinal lymphadenopathy. The heart size is normal. There is no pleural, soft tissue or bony abnormality.

In summary, there are multiple small, calcified lung nodules with no other radiographic findings of note. If the patient is well, this would most likely be due to a previous episode of **Varicella zoster virus** pneumonia. If the patient is unwell, I would consider metastatic disease. Silicosis would be a less likely cause, as the nodules are diffuse and the hilar nodes are not calcified.

To take this further, I would review any previous imaging and correlate the findings with the clinical history, looking for previous admissions for pneumonia associated with chickenpox infection. If this is an incidental finding in an asymptomatic patient, it would not require follow-up.

Discussion

For most classical chest radiology viva cases, the lists of possible differential diagnoses can be long, and this is true for multiple calcified lung nodules. In the exam setting, the key to most chest cases is to identify the main abnormality, define the distribution and look for any associated findings. These factors should help you to refine your long differential list to a more sensible short list of possible diagnoses. The ability to do this is the key to both a successful viva exam and the skill of a good radiologist. If you blindly recite a long list of differentials in the viva, without thought, you run the risk of being quizzed on each and every condition you have mentioned. This is a situation to avoid at all costs. In your daily work, the long list would also be of no practical value to a clinician.

Healed VZV pneumonia is commonly seen in routine clinical practice and is often an incidental CXR finding. Histoplasmosis is rare in the United Kingdom but endemic in the United States. The finding of multiple small, calcified lung nodules is similar in both of these conditions. However, histoplasmosis is also associated with mediastinal nodal and splenic calcification as well as upper lobe fibrosis, which are not features of VZV infection.

A classic "Aunt Minnie" viva case comprises a CXR with multiple calcified lung nodules of varying sizes associated with a sclerotic or missing proximal humerus at the edge of the film. The unifying diagnosis is calcified osteosarcoma metastases.

Calcified lung metastases are commonly secondary to sarcoma, mucinous tumours of the colon or breast, papillary thyroid carcinoma, ovarian cystadenocarcinoma and testicular tumours.

Pearls

- To narrow the list of differential diagnoses, critically review whether there is/are: any calcified mediastinal nodes or upper lobe fibrosis (histoplasmosis/silicosis), an enlarged heart (mitral stenosis), bone abnormalities (current/previous sarcoma) or a superior mediastinal mass (thyroid cancer).
- Consider healed VZV pneumonia with multiple, small, well-defined nodules in the absence of any other radiographic findings.
- It is often helpful to subdivide differential diagnoses based on patient well-being, as this demonstrates knowledge and insight: "If the patient is clinically well, I would consider . . . If the patient is unwell, I would consider . . ."

7

Large cavitating lung lesion

"CAT"

	Condition	Associated features
C	Cancer (primary more than secondary)	Primary – more commonly solitary Metastases – more commonly multiple Lymphangitis carcinomatosis Hilar/mediastinal lymphadenopathy Rib lesions: sclerotic or lytic Previous surgery: mastectomy, axillary clips, oesophageal stent, cervical clips Thick- or thin-walled
A	Abscess	Usually a single cavitating lesion Thick-walled Air-fluid level Lower lobe predominance – suggests aspiration
T	TB (reactivation)	Most commonly posterior segments of the upper lobe and apical segment of the lower lobe Other lung masses/nodules Often bilateral Cavity may contain an air-fluid level May be surrounded by consolidation "Tree-in-bud" nodularity on CT Sometimes pleural effusion Lymphadenopathy rare

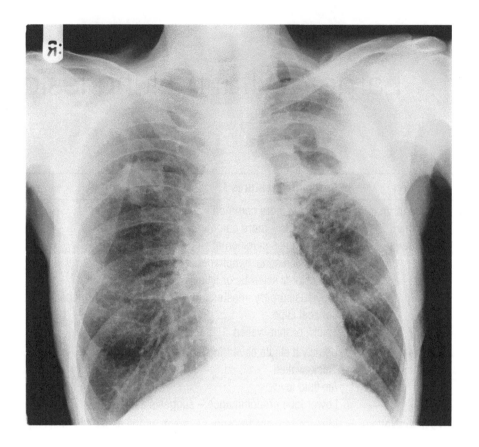

Diagnosis: Reactivation TB

MODEL ANSWER

This is a frontal chest radiograph of an adult male patient.

There is a large cavitating lesion within the left upper lobe. There is no air-fluid level within it. There is consolidation adjacent to the cavity, more pronounced inferiorly and laterally.

There is a further smaller mass within the right upper zone with a well-defined irregular outline. This lesion may also contain a small cavity in its medial aspect but is predominantly solid.

There is a generalised coarsening of the interstitial lung markings in the remainder of the lungs. The heart size is normal. There is no hilar lymphadenopathy and no destructive bony lesion.

In summary, there is a large cavitating lesion within the left upper lobe and a smaller mass in the right upper zone. The most likely causes include reactivation TB, advanced primary squamous cell carcinoma of the lung and lung abscesses.

To take this further, I would review the clinical history and arrange for a CT scan of the chest for clarification.

(The CT scans of the chest are then shown.)

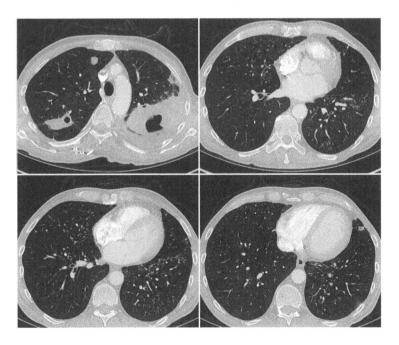

These are selected axial contrast-enhanced CT images of the chest, displayed on lung windows. The two large cavitating lesions are again seen, lying in the posterior segments of both upper lobes.

There are further smaller nodules seen in both lungs. The lesion in the lingula of the left upper lobe also has a small cavity.

There is "tree-in-bud" nodularity within the middle lobe and left lower lobe.

No destructive bony lesion or lymphadenopathy can be seen.

The finding of bilateral upper lobe cavitatory lesions, in addition to a "tree-in-bud" pattern on CT, is suggestive of reactivation TB. The presence of cavitation in reactivation TB implies that the condition is highly contagious. Therefore, based on the radiological findings alone, the patient should be cared for in isolation. I would urgently inform the on-call chest physician and arrange for admission for isolation and antimicrobial therapy.

Discussion

The differential for a large cavitating lung mass contains the conditions seen in the mnemonic for multiple pulmonary nodules (*see* Case 4). However, it is rarer for lung metastases, Wegener's granulomatosis, rheumatoid nodules and septic emboli to produce this appearance. The three main causes of cavitating lung lesions (as listed in the table) cannot be reliably distinguished on CXR and it is sensible to recommend a CT scan for further evaluation to narrow the list of differential diagnoses.

In this case, the findings of bilateral upper lobe cavitation, involving the posterior segments of the upper lobes along with a "tree-in-bud" pattern, suggest reactivation TB. The "tree-in-bud" pattern is only seen on CT. The appearance is of centrilobular nodularity connecting to branching linear structures. It is typical when TB involves the airways (endobronchial spread) and suggests active infectious TB. Lymphadenopathy is not a feature of reactivation TB. Primary TB is characterised by consolidation without cavitation, hilar/mediastinal lymphadenopathy, pleural effusions and, sometimes, a miliary pattern of disease (*see* Case 5).

Primary lung tumours are more frequently solitary. Squamous cell carcinoma is the most common primary lung tumour to cavitate. This tumour is usually centrally located. If the tumour causes central bronchial obstruction, there is likely to be associated post-obstructive collapse/consolidation. Lobar collapse has well-recognised features which are unique to each lobe – such as Golden's S sign in the right upper lobe. These should be committed to memory as these cases are often used as "starter" films in the exam viva. When apical and peripheral, squamous cell carcinoma is also the tumour most commonly associated with Pancoast's syndrome.

Lung metastases are more commonly multiple. Those that have a propensity to cavitate include squamous cell carcinoma (nasopharyngeal, oesophageal and cervical), adenocarcinoma from the colon, melanoma and rarely sarcoma.

Pearls

- A large cavitating mass in the upper lobe is likely to be reactivation TB or a primary lung tumour.
- If there are bilateral upper lobe abnormalities, TB is favoured.
- Ask for a CT scan for further evaluation.
- "Tree-in-bud" nodularity is suggestive of endobronchial spread of TB.
- If you suspect active TB, recommend urgent referral to a chest physician for admission, isolation and antimicrobial therapy.

8.
Anterior mediastinal mass

"Four T's"

Condition	Associated features
Thymic mass	Pleural metastases if malignant
Teratoma (germ cell tumour)	Younger age Often contain fat and enhancing septa on CT Calcification – rim or teeth/bone fragments
Thyroid (retrosternal)	Continuity with neck and superior mediastinum Deviation of the trachea
Terrible lymphoma	Lymphadenopathy in middle and posterior mediastinum as well as axilla, neck, abdomen and pelvis Splenomegaly

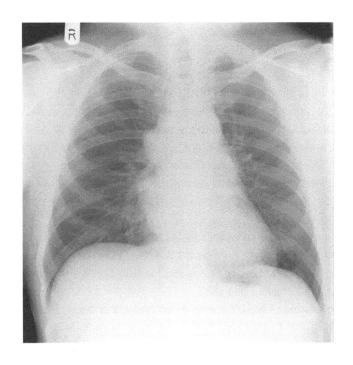

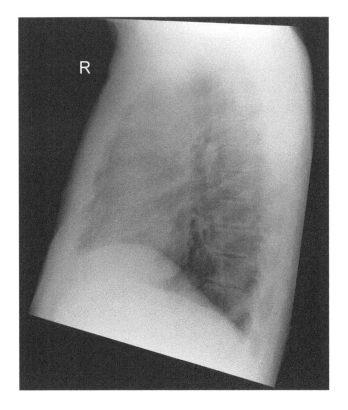

Diagnosis: Malignant thymoma with pleural metastases

MODEL ANSWER

This is a frontal and right lateral chest radiograph of an adult patient. There is a lobulated right-sided mediastinal mass, which forms a wide angle with the adjacent lung parenchyma. It effaces the ascending aorta as well as the right heart border. On the lateral radiograph, there is increased density within the retrosternal clear space. These features all confirm an anterior location.

There are several well-defined ovoid opacities projected over the peripheral right lung. The left lung is clear. The hila are clearly seen and are normal. No bony abnormality can be seen.

In summary, there is an anterior mediastinal mass with several opacities in the right hemithorax. The most likely cause is a thymic tumour with possible pleural metastases. The differential diagnoses include lymphoma and germ cell tumours. A thyroid mass seems less likely.

To take this further, I would obtain a contrast-enhanced CT scan of the chest and arrange for this to be discussed in the next thoracic MDT [multidisciplinary team] meeting.

Discussion

The boundaries of the anterior mediastinum are the sternum anteriorly, pleura laterally and the anterior aspect of the trachea and posterior margin of the heart posteriorly.

The anterior mediastinum contains lymph nodes, the thymus, the heart and the ascending aorta. An enlarged retrosternal thyroid gland can lie in the superior part of the anterior mediastinum, and will be continuous with the neck.

On a frontal CXR, a mediastinal mass will efface the normal mediastinal contents within the same compartment. This will result in the loss of the anatomical edge normally visible on the CXR (or, to put it another way, it will create a silhouette sign). For example, if the ascending aorta is effaced, the mass must lie within the anterior mediastinum. If the contents are not effaced, the mass does not lie within that compartment; for example, if hilar vessels are seen projected through a mass, it cannot lie within the middle mediastinum and must be located either anteriorly or posteriorly.

The majority of anterior mediastinal masses are lymphoid or thymic in origin. These conditions can be more easily differentiated on CT than CXR. Extensive lymphadenopathy in other distant locations suggests lymphoma. Pleural metastases can be suggestive of a thymic tumour. A tumour of germ cell origin (teratoma) often contains fat, calcifications and enhancing septations.

The age of the patient can be an important discriminator. Germ cell tumours are more prevalent in younger people, while thymic tumours affect older adults. Lymphoma can affect any age group.

Pearls

- A mediastinal mass forms an obtuse angle with the adjacent lung parenchyma.
- Look for effacement of heart borders and ascending aorta to confirm an anterior location.
- On a CT scan, look at the pleura for deposits (thymoma), lymphadenopathy outside the anterior mediastinum (lymphoma), a mass containing fat and enhancing septations (germ cell tumour).
- Mention the visibility of hilar vessels through the mass (hilum overlay sign) indicating no middle mediastinal component.
- Consider an enlarged thyroid if the mass lies superiorly and shows contiguity with the neck.
- Try to establish the patient's age to narrow the list of differential diagnoses: germ cell tumour = younger person; thymic tumour = older person.
- CT is required for further characterisation and to plan a possible percutaneous biopsy.
- MDT discussion is essential.

9

Pleural lesions

"METAL"

	Condition	Associated features
M	Mesothelioma	Pleural effusion (often large and unilateral) Pleural thickening, which may be multifocal or circumferential Often involves the mediastinal pleura and interlobar fissures Ipsilateral volume loss Calcified pleural plaques (previous asbestos exposure) Chest wall invasion
E	Empyema	Pleural fluid with locules of gas Pleural thickening and enhancement Smooth margin, convex towards the lung "Split pleura" sign Adjacent pneumonia
T	Thymic tumour (invasive thymoma or thymic carcinoma)	Anterior mediastinal mass with lobulated contour Encases mediastinal structures Spreads along pleural surfaces Unilateral nodular pleural thickening
A	Adenocarcinoma metastases	Evidence of metastatic disease: • lymphadenopathy • lymphangitis carcinomatosis • bone lesions • lung nodules/masses • pleural effusion

	Condition	Associated features
L	Lymphoma Loculated pleural effusion	Lymphoma: • variable – solitary nodule or diffuse pleural thickening • pleural effusion • bilateral asymmetrical hilar enlargement • consolidation • lung nodules/masses • lymphangitis carcinomatosis Loculated pleural effusion: • localised pleural fluid • smooth margin, concave towards the lung • no pleural thickening or enhancement

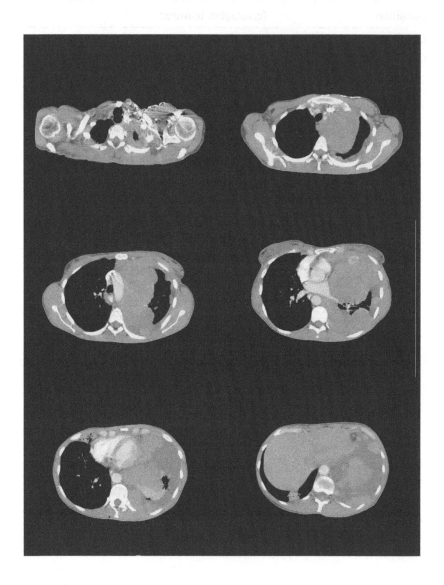

Diagnosis: Invasive thymoma with pleural metastases

MODEL ANSWER

These are selected contrast-enhanced CT images of the chest in an adult, displayed on soft tissue windows.

There is a large soft tissue mass encasing the left hemithorax. The mass invades the left side of the mediastinum and is seen on these images to encase the aortic arch, descending aorta and the left pulmonary vein. There is mediastinal shift to the right. The mediastinal mass is continuous with and enlarges the pleural space. The pleural mass has a lobulated inner contour. There are no areas of pleural calcification. The pleural mass has caused volume loss of the left lung, and there is compressive atelectasis in the base of the left lower lobe. There is a left pleural effusion. No discrete lung mass is seen. There is no bony abnormality – in particular, there is no rib erosion adjacent to the pleural mass.

In summary, there is an extensive mass in the left hemithorax that invades the mediastinum and left pleural space, and encases the great vessels. This is most likely neoplastic. The most likely cause is a thymic tumour, mesothelioma or adenocarcinoma metastases.

To take this further, I would review this scan on lung and bone windows to look for any evidence of lung nodules or skeletal lesions to indicate metastases. I would like to know about any history of smoking and asbestos exposure. I would review any relevant previous imaging. The patient should be discussed at the next chest MDT meeting, with a view to CT or ultrasound-guided biopsy of the mass for histology.

Discussion

Pleural masses form an obtuse angle with the chest wall. The presence of circumferential pleural thickening, pleural thickening greater than 1 cm in depth, widespread pleural nodularity and involvement of the mediastinal pleura are all features associated with malignancy. However, definitive differentiation of benign from malignant lesions will almost certainly require a biopsy.

Aggressive thymic tumours, mesothelioma and metastases are often indistinguishable on a CT image. It would be sensible to mention these three diagnoses in cases involving multiple pleural masses or extensive pleural thickening. In this case, the additional presence of a large mediastinal mass suggests invasive thymoma with pleural involvement. Pleural metastatic disease is most commonly secondary to lung or breast cancer, signs of which may be visible on the available chest imaging.

Malignant mesothelioma is strongly associated with previous exposure to asbestos, but not all people exposed to asbestos will develop mesothelioma (approximately 5%). The latent period between exposure and development of this condition is between 30 and 45 years.

A rare, mostly benign cause of a solitary pleural lesion is a pleural fibroma. This is commonly a large, smooth, spherical mass, which may be pedunculated and mobile within the pleural space. It is usually asymptomatic, but there is an association with hypertrophic osteoarthropathy (HOA). It is a condition to remember when confronted with a large pleural mass on CXR or CT.

Empyema and transudative pleural effusions are most easily distinguished on contrast-enhanced CT imaging. Empyema is commonly unilateral, adjacent to an area of pneumonia/consolidation and can form a convex border with the lung (lentiform shape). The "split pleura" sign of empyema refers to thickening and enhancement of the visceral and parietal pleura, separated by the purulent fluid. The adjacent soft tissue of the chest wall may also display signs of inflammation, such as thickening and stranding of the fat.

As with most oncology cases, in both the examination (viva and long case) and in practice, MDT discussion and consideration of image-guided biopsy are sensible management steps (the possible exceptions are hepatocellular carcinoma (HCC), in which classical magnetic resonance imaging [MRI] findings are sufficient to make the diagnosis, and sarcoma, in which referral to a specialist centre is often preferred before biopsy).

Pearls

- In contrast to lung masses, which form a narrow (acute) angle, pleural and mediastinal masses form an obtuse angle with the chest wall.
- Lung and breast carcinoma are the tumours responsible for the majority of pleural metastases – scrutinise the available images for evidence of mastectomy or primary lung tumour.

- Look for a dominant anterior mediastinal mass and invasion of the mediastinal fat in aggressive thymic tumours.
- Look for pleural calcification and ipsilateral volume loss in mesothelioma.
- For pleural fluid, look for the signs to distinguish between infected or simple collections.

10.
Hyperlucent hemithorax

"CPAP"

	Cause	Associated features
C	Chest wall (Poland's syndrome, polio, mastectomy)	Asymmetry of thoracic wall soft tissues Poland's syndrome: rib/scapula hypoplasia, absent pectoralis major, associated with ipsilateral breast aplasia Polio: ipsilateral scapula/humeral hypoplasia Mastectomy: surgical clips in the ipsilateral axilla may also be seen
P	Positioning (rotation/ scoliosis)	Asymmetry of the distance between the spinous processes and medial ends of the clavicles (this may be due to poor radiographic technique or an unwell patient who cannot be adequately positioned) Patients with thoracic scoliosis may have an inherent anatomical rotation
A	Airways disease (airway obstruction, emphysema, Swyer–James' syndrome, congenital lobar emphysema)	All: expiratory air trapping; this may result in increased ipsilateral lung volume and contralateral mediastinal shift (the exception being Swyer–James' syndrome) Swyer–James' syndrome: normal or small volume lung with small ipsilateral hilar vessels Foreign body: • commonly seen in young children/toddlers • occasional radio-opaque foreign body seen in the ipsilateral bronchus Congenital lobar emphysema: • babies/early childhood • hyperinflated lobe of lung

	Cause	Associated features
P	Pneumothorax Pulmonary embolus (PE)	Pneumothorax: • lung edge visible • absence of lung markings peripherally • always comment on mediastinal shift and a possible tension pneumothorax PE: • enlarged ipsilateral central pulmonary artery with paucity of the peripheral pulmonary vasculature • peripheral lung opacities (infarcts) • pleural effusion

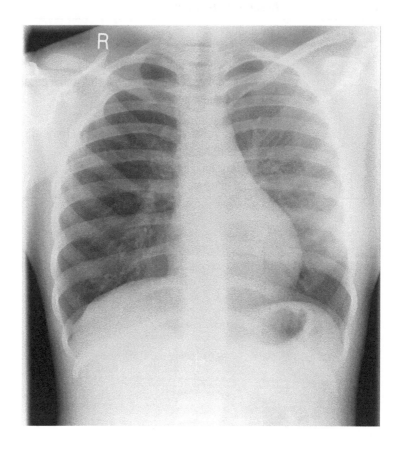

Diagnosis: Poland's syndrome

Definition: Hyperlucency of one lung

MODEL ANSWER

This is a frontal chest radiograph of an adult female. There is hyperlucency of the right hemithorax. The film is well centred with no evidence of rotation. The lungs are clear, with equal and normal lung volumes. The hilar vessels and pulmonary vasculature are normal. The pleural spaces are clear. No pneumothorax can be seen.

There is a decreased amount of soft tissue in the right thoracic wall. The right breast shadow is absent, but there are no associated right axillary surgical clips. The right third rib and scapula are hypoplastic.

In summary, there is a hyperlucent right hemithorax. This is most likely related to the decreased soft tissue overlying the right chest wall. The skeletal features are suggestive of Poland's syndrome. A right mastectomy is also a possibility, but this seems less likely given that the patient appears to be a young adult and there are no surgical clips demonstrated in the axilla.

To take this further, I would review any previous imaging to assess if the hyperlucent right hemithorax is a constant feature. A clinical examination could be performed to assess for the absence of the right pectoralis major, hypoplasia of the breast or evidence of syndactyly, to confirm the diagnosis of Poland's syndrome. If there were any clinical doubt, a non-contrast CT of the chest could be performed to further assess the musculature.

Discussion

This case allows the examiner to test your ability to work through a set of differential diagnoses and to justify which you think is the most likely diagnosis. The provided mnemonic will get you out of trouble if your mind goes blank; however, an alternative approach to this case (once you have spotted the unilateral hyperlucent hemithorax) is to work anatomically from outside in, and to assess the structures as you go.

Before launching into your description of the hyperlucent hemithorax, take a second to ensure the abnormality is not within the more radio-opaque hemithorax. Good examples of this would include a pleural effusion on a supine film, unilateral pleural thickening and unilateral consolidation.

Patient rotation is a common cause of a unilateral hyperlucent hemithorax. If the patient is rotated to the right, the projected distance between the medial end of the right clavicle and the spinous processes will be increased, and the right hemithorax will be hyperlucent.

Poland's syndrome is the congenital absence of the pectoralis major muscle. It is a popular exam case. Recognised associations include rib, scapula and upper limb hypoplasia as well as syndactyly (fusion of the digits). Clinical examination should be sufficient to establish the diagnosis, but CT will unequivocally confirm the abnormality. The patient may have a breast implant for cosmesis.

Air trapping is a feature of airway obstruction and results in hyperexpansion. It is effectively demonstrated on a CXR taken during expiration. The affected lung will not reduce in volume (as the air is trapped). If the problem affects only one lung, there may be contralateral mediastinal shift as the normal lung deflates.

Swyer–James' syndrome occurs as a result of viral bronchiolitis in infancy, which disrupts the normal development of the lung. It is asymptomatic and often diagnosed as an incidental finding in adulthood. It is characterised by a hyperlucent lung with expiratory air trapping and reduced hilar and pulmonary vascularity. The lung is usually of small volume.

Foreign body inhalation is commonly seen in children with a relevant acute history. The air trapping occurs due to a ball-valve effect of the foreign body in the bronchus. The foreign body is not always radio-opaque – an inhaled peanut is a good example of this.

A large central pulmonary embolus can obstruct blood flow to the peripheral pulmonary veins. The resultant paucity of the peripheral pulmonary vascular markings creates the appearance of a hyperlucent lung, the Westermark sign. However, this is rarely seen in PE. Other recognised CXR findings of acute PE include peripheral wedge-shaped opacities due to pulmonary infarction (Hampton's hump), pleural effusion and an enlarged pulmonary artery.

Pearls

- First establish whether the image shows unilateral hyperlucency or unilateral increased opacity.
- Look at the medial clavicles for signs of rotation, then look at the soft tissues of the neck, lateral chest wall and breast shadows for asymmetry (Poland's syndrome, mastectomy, polio).
- Assess and describe lung volume (Swyer–James' syndrome) and hilar size (enlarged pulmonary artery in PE).
- Does the contralateral lung appear normal? If it is reduced in volume and the hyperlucent lung is expanded, consider contralateral lung agenesis/hypoplasia.
- If there is the possibility of airway obstruction, ask to see further imaging to look for air trapping, either an expiratory CXR or HRCT with expiratory images.
- Remember the inhaled peanut/foreign body in paediatric cases.

11.
Completely opacified hemithorax

"Every CXR Aids Patient Management"

	Condition	Associated features
E	Effusion	Tracheal deviation/mediastinal shift to the contralateral side If secondary to malignancy – contralateral lung nodules, mastectomy, nodal enlargement, rib lesions
C	Consolidation Collapse	Consolidation: ● air bronchograms ● no tracheal deviation Collapse: ● tracheal deviation/mediastinal shift to the ipsilateral side ● check endotracheal tube position – is it too near the carina or in the right main bronchus? ● if secondary to central obstructing tumour/metastasis – assess for contralateral lung nodules, mastectomy, nodal enlargement, rib lesions
A	Agenesis	Tracheal deviation to ipsilateral side No change compared with previous CXRs (if available)
P	Pneumonectomy	Tracheal deviation to ipsilateral side Fifth/sixth rib excision or signs of thoracotomy Surgical clips
M	Mesothelioma	Calcified pleural plaques Pleural effusion Limited mediastinal shift due to encasement of the lung

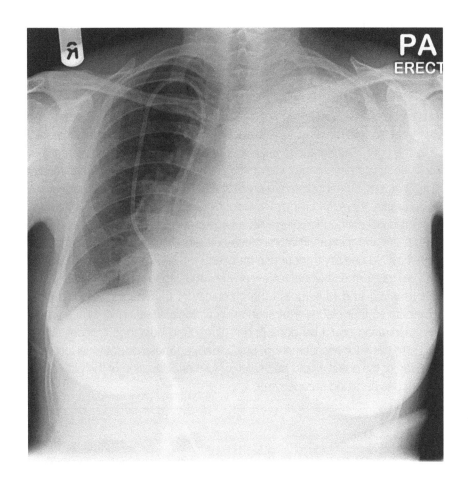

Diagnosis: Malignant pleural effusion (secondary to metastatic osteosarcoma)

MODEL ANSWER

This is a frontal chest radiograph of a young adult female patient. There is a completely opacified left hemithorax with tracheal deviation and moderate mediastinal shift to the right. The right lung is clear. There is a tunnelled right internal jugular central venous catheter in situ, with its tip at the junction of the superior vena cava and right atrium. Both breasts are present and there is no bony abnormality.

In summary, there is complete whiteout of the left hemithorax with contralateral mediastinal shift, in keeping with a large pleural effusion. The presence of a Hickman line and a large unilateral pleural effusion is suggestive of an underlying malignancy. No primary tumour can be seen.

To take this further, I would review any previous imaging to identify any known primary tumour and to establish the chronicity of the effusion. I would contact the clinician so that pleural aspiration and cytological tests might be performed. Pleural aspiration could be done under ultrasound guidance if necessary. This would also allow for assessment of any underlying mass or potential loculations. A CT scan of the chest would be useful for further evaluation of the pleura, mediastinal nodes and lung parenchyma.

Discussion

The completely opacified hemithorax is reasonably common in normal clinical practice. Such opacification is referred to as "whiteout" on a chest radiograph. There are a limited number of causes. The main factor to consider in narrowing the list of differential diagnoses is whether there is any mediastinal shift; if so, in which direction is this?

In this case, there is contralateral mediastinal shift indicating that the underlying cause of the whiteout is expanding the affected hemithorax. The whiteout is therefore not due to lung collapse, lung agenesis or a pneumonectomy, all of which result in ipsilateral volume loss. The underlying cause is most likely to be a large unilateral pleural effusion. These are strongly associated with malignancy, and the presence of a Hickman line (used for chemotherapy) would support this diagnosis. If you suspect a malignant unilateral pleural effusion, you should scrutinise the film for evidence of a primary cancer and metastatic disease, especially in the ribs, shoulder girdle, mediastinum and contralateral lung. In this case, there was underlying osteosarcoma of the pelvis with pleural metastases and a large left pleural effusion, proven on CT.

Pearls

- Note the position of the trachea.
- Ipsilateral mediastinal shift is caused by lung collapse, pulmonary agenesis and pneumonectomy.
- In large unilateral pleural effusions, there may be contralateral or no mediastinal shift.
- Large unilateral pleural effusions are most often caused by malignancy.
- Common causes of malignant pleural effusions are lung and breast carcinoma, lymphoma and mesothelioma – look for evidence of bony and contralateral lung metastases.
- Mesothelioma may encase the lung, reducing the amount of mediastinal shift possible.
- Mention the need to review previous films.

12.
Peripheral consolidation

"AEIOU"

	Condition	Associated features
A	Alveolar sarcoidosis	Mid and upper zone distribution Bilateral symmetrical reticulonodular pattern Underlying nodules on CT – subpleural, fissural and bronchovascular distribution Mediastinal lymphadenopathy
E	Eosinophilic pneumonia (chronic)	Blood eosinophilia Nodules and reticular opacities uncommon Classically affects young adult females
I	Infarct	Wedge-shaped opacities Evidence of pulmonary embolus Pleural effusions
O	Cryptogenic Organising pneumonia (COP)	Patchy peripheral consolidation with associated "ground-glass" shadowing Predominantly lower zone Reticular opacities Nodules Classically affects 40–70 year olds
U	contUsion	History/evidence of trauma, e.g. rib fractures, pneumothorax, subcutaneous emphysema, aortic injury

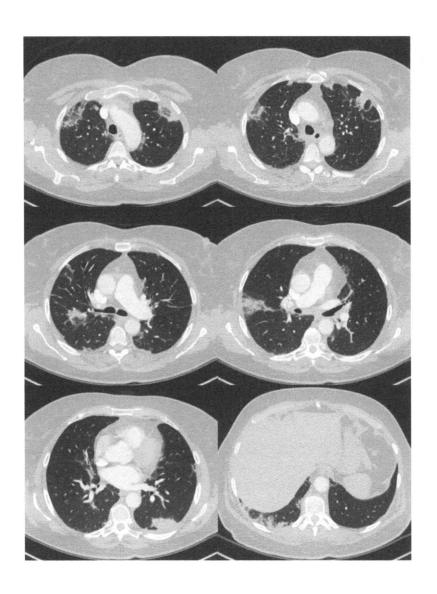

Diagnosis: COP

MODEL ANSWER

These are selected contrast-enhanced axial CT images of the thorax of an adult female patient, displayed on lung windows.

There are multiple bilateral foci of well-defined consolidation with surrounding "ground-glass" opacification in a subpleural distribution. There are several associated reticular opacities with some distortion of the surrounding lung parenchyma.

The lung volumes appear normal and symmetrical. No lung nodules or pleural effusions are visible. I can see no gross mediastinal lymphadenopathy or large pulmonary embolus on these images, however I would normally assess for these features on different window settings.

In summary, there are multiple areas of peripheral consolidation with associated "ground-glass" opacification. The most likely diagnosis is cryptogenic organising pneumonia. The differential diagnoses include eosinophilic pneumonia and atypical sarcoidosis. With a history or evidence of pulmonary embolus or thoracic trauma, I would also include pulmonary infarction and contusion in this list.

To take this further, I would review any recent blood test results for eosinophilia. I would also review the patient's medical and drug history for collagen vascular disease or a recent change in medication. I would refer the patient to a chest physician for further management.

Discussion

COP is an inflammatory lung disease of unknown aetiology in 50% of cases. Known precipitants include the pulmonary manifestations of rheumatoid arthritis (RA), drug toxicity (e.g. amiodarone) and viral infections.

COP has a variable appearance but most often shows areas of consolidation and/or "ground-glass" opacification in a subpleural and peripheral distribution. Nodules, mass-like lesions and pleural thickening may also occur. The typical presentation is of worsening shortness of breath in a middle-aged patient that does not respond to antibiotics. There is usually an excellent response to steroids.

Chronic eosinophilic pneumonia (CEP) is also characterised by bilateral peripheral consolidation. It is distinguished from COP by blood tests to assess for the presence of eosinophilia. The radiological appearances of both conditions are very similar. However, lung nodules and reticular opacities are less common in CEP. A tissue diagnosis is required for confirmation. CEP also responds quickly to treatment with steroids.

Pearls

- COP and CEP can be indistinguishable on CT. Mention both in your list of differential diagnoses.
- Pulmonary sarcoidosis is the great mimic. It can therefore be considered in most pulmonary exam cases.
- Assess the pulmonary artery and branches for filling defects.
- Check the ribs for signs of trauma.

13.
Diffuse bilateral consolidation

"HARPIE"

	Condition	Associated features
H	Heart failure Pulmonary haemorrhage	Heart failure: cardiac enlargement
A	Acute respiratory distress syndrome (ARDS)	
R	Reaction to drugs	
P	Pneumocystis pneumonia (PCP)	Pleural effusion and hilar lymphadenopathy are uncommon
I	non-specific Interstitial pneumonia (NSIP)	
E	EAA	

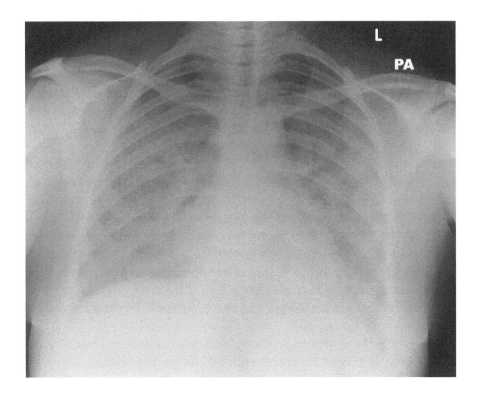

Diagnosis: PCP

MODEL ANSWER

This is a frontal chest radiograph of an adult female patient. There is diffuse bilateral increased density in both lungs with a middle and lower zone predominance. The pleural spaces are clear. The cardiomediastinal contour is normal. There is no bony abnormality.

In summary, there is diffuse bilateral lung consolidation. This is a non-specific finding for which there are many possible causes. These include both cardiogenic and non-cardiogenic pulmonary oedema, drug reactions, pulmonary haemorrhage, PCP and interstitial lung diseases such as NSIP and EAA.

To take this further, I would review the patient history and recent imaging to establish chronicity. I would like to know if there is a history of immunosuppression to suggest a diagnosis of PCP, or severe illness or recent trauma to suggest a diagnosis of ARDS. Is there a recent history of cytotoxic drug use or change of medication? Is there a history of repeated exposure to an allergen to suggest EAA?

If the clinical history does not indicate a specific diagnosis, an HRCT scan of the chest may help to further characterise the pattern of disease.

Discussion

No features on this radiograph clearly indicate the diagnosis. Patient history is very important, particularly any immunosuppression, recent trauma or severe illness, new medications and exposure to allergens. The patient in this case was HIV positive.

A case of cardiogenic pulmonary oedema may seem too easy for the exam, but it would be silly to miss this diagnosis if it were presented. In the presence of cardiomegaly, be sure to check for the classic signs of upper lobe blood diversion, bronchial cuffing, Kerley's A and B lines and pleural effusions.

ARDS can be due to a direct or indirect insult to the lung, such as severe pneumonia and aspiration, or systemic sepsis, trauma, burns and drug overdoses. The chest radiograph may be normal for the first 12–24 hours after the onset of symptoms, with widespread bilateral symmetrical consolidation developing during days 1 to 5 of the condition.

PCP is an opportunistic infection in the immunocompromised, including those with HIV/AIDS, on chemotherapy or post-transplant patients. The pattern seen on CXR is initially of bilateral symmetrical perihilar opacification rapidly progressing to diffuse bilateral consolidation. Hilar lymphadenopathy and pleural effusions are rare.

NSIP commonly presents with bilateral lower zone reticular opacities. HRCT reveals associated "ground-glass" opacification (GGO).

EAA is caused by repeated exposure to organic particulate antigens. Typical sufferers are farmworkers and people who keep birds. Subacute EAA is characterised by bilateral symmetrical nodular opacities and GGO, sparing the bases.

HRCT findings may help to narrow the list of differential diagnoses.

- Pulmonary oedema appears as perihilar and lower zone GGO, smooth septal thickening and often pleural effusions.
- PCP has variable appearances. It may appear as diffuse or perihilar GGO, focal septal thickening and thin-walled cysts, which may lead to pneumothoraces.
- NSIP appears as subpleural GGO with irregular linear or reticular opacities and small nodules, with subpleural cysts in advanced cases. There is a lower zone predominance.
- EAA shows as centrilobular nodules, extensive GGO and air trapping that spares the lower zones.

Pearls

- Diffuse bilateral consolidation is a non-specific finding.
- The patient history is important and relevant.
- HRCT can narrow the list of differential diagnoses.
- This mnemonic also applies to GGO on HRCT.
- In the clinical setting of immunosuppression, the findings of diffuse consolidation on CXR or diffuse GGO on HRCT are both highly suggestive of PCP.

14.
Bilateral hilar enlargement

"SLIPS"

	Condition	Associated features
S	Sarcoidosis	Lobulated symmetrical hilar enlargement with right paratracheal stripe widening due to lymphadenopathy – Garland's triad
		Reticulonodular opacities in the mid and upper zone
		Nodules along subpleural surfaces and bronchovascular bundles
		"Egg-shell" calcification of nodes
		Upper zone fibrosis and traction bronchiectasis in end-stage disease
L	Lymphoma	Bilateral but asymmetrical hilar enlargement
		Enlarged hilar nodes usually abut the cardiac borders
I	Infection (especially viral, TB)	Unilateral or bilateral hilar lymphadenopathy with variable consolidation
		Bilateral hilar enlargement is rare in TB
P	Pulmonary artery hypertension (PAH)	Enlarged main pulmonary artery
		Enlarged left and right pulmonary arteries
		Mural calcification of pulmonary arteries in long-standing severe PAH
		Decreased peripheral vascular markings ("pruning")
		Cardiomegaly (especially right ventricle)
		Lung parenchymal abnormalities, e.g. fibrosis, emphysema
S	Small cell lung carcinoma	Non-specific
		Unilateral or asymmetrical hilar and/or mediastinal lymphadenopathy
		Primary tumour may not be apparent

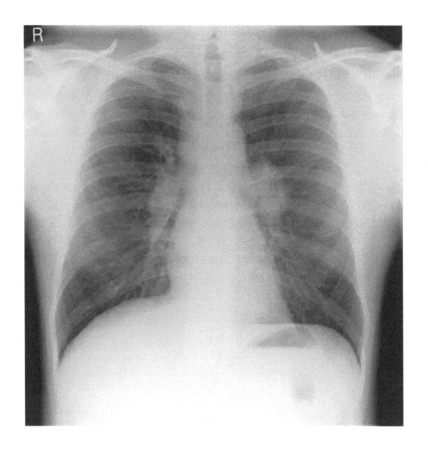

Diagnosis: Pulmonary sarcoidosis

MODEL ANSWER

This is a frontal chest radiograph of an adult male patient. There is bilateral symmetrical hilar enlargement with an associated widening of the right paratracheal stripe. This is due to lymphadenopathy. The pulmonary arteries are of normal calibre. The heart is of normal size. The lungs and pleural spaces are clear. No bony abnormality is evident.

In summary, the features of bilateral symmetrical hilar and right paratracheal lymphadenopathy are typical of sarcoidosis.

I would compare these findings with any relevant previous imaging and consider HRCT of the chest, if not previously performed, to assess for subpleural, perifissural and bronchovascular nodules. The patient should be referred to the chest physicians for further management.

Discussion

Hilar enlargement is either due to hilar lymphadenopathy or enlargement of the pulmonary arteries. It can be difficult to reliably distinguish between these two pathologies on CXR. Lobulated hilar enlargement is more suggestive of lymphadenopathy, whereas smooth hilar enlargement with peripheral decreased vascular markings suggests PAH.

The classical pattern of lymphadenopathy in sarcoidosis is of symmetrical bilateral hilar and right paratracheal nodal enlargement (Garland's triad). Anterior and posterior mediastinal nodal involvement is rare. Patients may also have associated lung parenchymal abnormalities, which are better appreciated on HRCT. Typical findings include small subpleural, perifissural and peribronchovascular nodules distributed in the mid and upper zones. However, sarcoidosis is the great mimic, and has many associated but atypical appearances. There may be upper lobe fibrosis in advanced disease.

PAH may be primary (idiopathic) or secondary to cardiac (e.g. left-to-right shunt), lung parenchymal (e.g. interstitial fibrosis, emphysema) or vascular abnormalities (chronic pulmonary embolic disease). Therefore, once you have decided that the pulmonary arteries are enlarged, always look for any evidence suggesting an underlying cause. CT is essential to further evaluate the pulmonary vessels and lung parenchyma. PAH can be diagnosed when the main pulmonary artery is greater than 29 mm in diameter and/or is larger than the adjacent ascending aorta.

Severe dilatation of the central pulmonary arteries with "pruning" of the peripheral pulmonary arteries (i.e. the peripheral arteries are not seen) are the classical CXR findings of Eisenmenger's syndrome. In this condition there is an underlying left-to-right cardiac shunt, such as an atrial septal defect, ventricular septal defect or patent ductus arteriosus. As a reaction to many years of increased pulmonary blood flow, the peripheral pulmonary vascular resistance increases (through reactive muscular hypertrophy and endothelial thickening) resulting in "pruning", PAH, reversal of flow in the cardiac shunt and cyanosis.

Pearls

- To narrow the list of differential diagnoses in bilateral hilar enlargement on CXR, assess the shape and symmetry of the hila as well as the peripheral vascularity of the lungs.
- Lobulated hilar enlargement with normal peripheral vasculature suggests hilar lymphadenopathy.
- Smooth hilar enlargement with abrupt tapering of vessels suggests pulmonary artery enlargement.
- Sarcoidosis is the commonest cause of bilateral symmetric hilar enlargement.
- On HRCT, the presence of small nodules along the fissures is strongly suggestive of sarcoidosis.
- PAH may be primary (idiopathic) or secondary to lung, cardiac or thromboembolic pathology.

15.
Inferior rib notching

"AVN"

	Condition	Associated features
A	Arterial obstruction (Aortic coarctation, Blalock–Taussig shunt, Takayasu's arteritis)	Coarctation: • commonly bilateral, third to ninth ribs • abnormal aortic contour – prominent ascending and small descending aorta • cardiomegaly with or without pulmonary oedema • "figure 3" sign on CXR Blalock–Taussig shunt: • a procedure for the treatment of Tetralogy of Fallot (subclavian-pulmonary artery anastomosis) • unilateral rib notching on the side of procedure – upper three or four ribs • thoracotomy/median sternotomy wires • abnormal cardiac contour Takayasu's arteritis: unilateral rib notching on side of subclavian artery occlusion – most commonly left
V	Venous obstruction: superior vena cava obstruction	Rarely seen Evidence of malignancy (especially lung carcinoma, lymphoma) Superior mediastinal widening Hilar masses Lung nodules/masses Lytic rib lesions (metastases) Reticulonodular shadowing (lymphangitis)
N	Nerve (neurofibromatosis) Normal variant	Neurofibromatosis: • large notches (from intercostal neurofibromas) • if severe, very thin attenuated "ribbon" ribs (from pressure effects and rib dysplasia) • subcutaneous nodules • posterior mediastinal masses • kyphoscoliosis • interstitial lung disease with normal/increased volumes

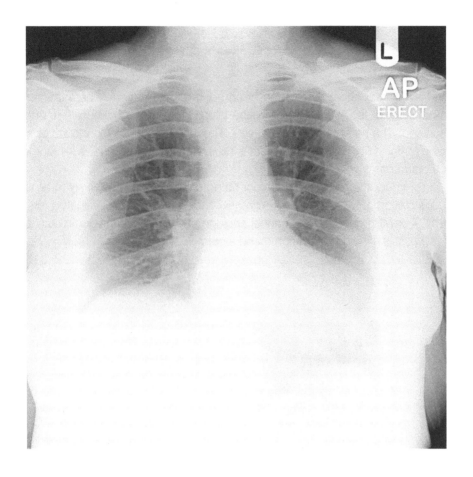

Diagnosis: Coarctation of the aorta

MODEL ANSWER

This is a frontal chest radiograph of an adult female patient. There is inferior rib notching of the fourth to eighth ribs bilaterally. The aortic knuckle is poorly visualised. The heart is of a normal size. The lungs are clear. No pleural or soft tissue abnormality is apparent. There is no evidence of previous cardiac surgery or thoracotomy.

In summary, there is bilateral inferior rib notching. This is most likely to be due to coarctation of the aorta. If this is a new finding, it could be evaluated further with CT or MR [magnetic resonance] angiography to assess the aortic arch and great vessels. I would also recommend a cardiology referral.

Discussion

"Would your diagnosis change if the rib notching was unilateral?"

"Er, no."

"Do you know any other causes of rib notching?"

"Er . . . er . . . idiopathic . . . um . . . no."

A case showing inferior rib notching will most likely be due to coarctation of the aorta. Most candidates will recognise this. As such, this case is not used to discriminate between more capable and less capable exam candidates. To test the depth of your knowledge, the examiner may question you on the underlying mechanism of rib notching, the differential diagnoses, the significance of unilateral rib notching in coarctation and the difference between the underlying pathologies in superior and inferior rib notching.

Inferior rib notching occurs due to the abnormal enlargement of either the intercostal artery, vein or nerve, all of which lie in the costal groove. The intercostal arteries become enlarged in the presence of a thoracic aortic stenosis or obstruction. Collateral blood flow bypasses the obstruction via the subclavian, internal mammary and third to ninth intercostal arteries, to reach the descending aorta. Therefore, inferior rib notching in aortic coarctation only affects the third to ninth ribs. The first and second intercostal arteries do not connect to the descending aorta, and the tenth to twelfth intercostal arteries do not connect to the subclavian artery.

The most common site of aortic coarctation is typically distal to the origin of the left subclavian artery (post-ductal). This causes raised blood pressure in both subclavian arteries and the development of bilateral collateral circulations, leading to bilateral inferior rib notching. If the aortic coarctation lies proximal to the origin of the left subclavian artery (pre-ductal), there will be post-stenotic low blood pressure in the left subclavian artery and pre-stenotic high blood pressure in the right subclavian artery, resulting in unilateral right-sided inferior rib notching. The anatomical situation in which unilateral left-sided inferior rib notching can occur is a little complex. However, if there is an aberrant right subclavian artery, the origin of which lies distal to a post-ductal aortic coarctation, unilateral left-sided rib notching will occur.

Inferior rib notching due to aortic coarctation is rare before the age of 6 years but is commonly seen in adults with this condition. The CXR may sometimes demonstrate a "figure 3" sign of the aortic contour. This appearance is due to pre-stenotic dilatation of the aortic knuckle and post-stenotic dilatation of the descending aorta, with the intervening narrow coarctation. Unfortunately, the "figure 3" sign is not a constant finding.

Deformed, thinned and irregular ribs ("ribbon" ribs) are associated with neurofibromatosis. This reflects both bone hypoplasia and the pressure effects of intercostal neurofibromas. "Ribbon" rib deformity is usually more pronounced than the inferior rib notching seen with coarctation. There may also be other associated features of neurofibromatosis, as described earlier in this case.

Superior rib notching is less common and has a separate list of differential diagnoses. It is sometimes seen in conditions producing resorption of bone, comparable to lateral clavicle resorption (*see* Case 23). Causes include RA, scleroderma, systemic lupus erythematosus and hyperparathyroidism.

Pearls

- Inferior rib notching is most likely due to coarctation of the aorta.
- In most cases, there is bilateral rib notching, with the focal aortic stenosis lying distal to the origin of the left subclavian artery.
- Unilateral rib notching occurs when there are differential pressures in the subclavian arteries.
- If the area of focal aortic stenosis lies proximal to the origin of the left subclavian artery, there will be unilateral right-sided rib notching.
- If there is an aberrant origin of the right subclavian artery, distal to the focal stenosis and the left subclavian artery origin, there will be unilateral left-sided rib notching.
- Coarctation of the aorta is associated with Turner's syndrome, berry aneurysms and a bicuspid aortic valve.
- If there is marked thinning of multiple ribs, with both superior and inferior rib notching, consider neurofibromatosis ("ribbon" ribs).

Section 2

Musculoskeletal

16.
Diffuse osteosclerosis

"ROMPS"

	Condition	Associated features
R	Renal osteodystrophy	Occurs in children or adults "Rugger jersey" spine (ill-defined bands of endplate sclerosis) Subperiosteal bone resorption Secondary signs of renal failure: • haemodialysis or peritoneal dialysis lines • vascular fistulae • vascular and soft tissue calcifications
O	Osteopetrosis	Paediatric onset *Very* dense bone "Sandwich" vertebrae (well-defined endplate sclerosis) Fractures Sclerotic mandible with supernumerary teeth Erlenmeyer flask deformity
M	Metastases Myelofibrosis	Metastases: • focal cortical destruction/lytic lesions • lung nodules • lymphangitis carcinomatosis • evidence of surgery, e.g. mastectomy, axillary clips Myelofibrosis: • onset typically in those aged >50 years • narrowed medullary cavity • hepatosplenomegaly/splenectomy (surgical clips)
P	Pyknodysostosis	Paediatric onset Fractures Hypoplastic sclerotic mandible Multiple wormian bones "Pencil-sharpened" distal phalanges

	Condition	Associated features
S	Sickle cell disease	"Codfish"/H-shaped vertebrae
		Avascular necrosis (AVN) humeral/femoral heads
		Gallstones
		Absent/atrophic calcified spleen
		Cardiomegaly

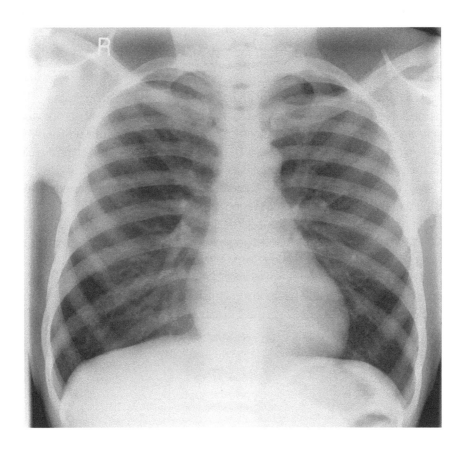

Diagnosis: Sickle cell disease

MODEL ANSWER

This is a frontal chest radiograph of an adult male patient. There is diffuse osteo-sclerosis throughout the bony skeleton. No associated osteolysis can be seen. There are central endplate depressions in multiple thoracic vertebral bodies, which have a biconcave shape, in keeping with H-shaped vertebrae. The lungs are clear and there is a normal cardiomediastinal contour.

In summary, there is diffuse osteosclerosis associated with H-shaped thoracic vertebrae. The findings suggest a diagnosis of sickle cell disease.

Other causes of diffuse osteosclerosis include sclerotic metastases, renal osteodystrophy, myelofibrosis and congenital conditions such as osteopetrosis. However, these diagnoses are less likely in this case.

If this is a new diagnosis, I would inform the requesting clinician and suggest referral of the patient to the haematology team for follow-up.

Discussion

Diffuse osteosclerosis is most likely to be demonstrated in the exam on a chest, abdominal or pelvic radiograph. Once you have decided that this is the key feature of the film, search for clues to distinguish between the different conditions.

The case shown is just one of several manifestations of sickle cell disease that can appear in an exam situation. Other diagnostic clues, which can appear individually or in combination, include:

- H-shaped or biconcave vertebrae without osteosclerosis
- an enlarged heart and pulmonary plethora due to high-output cardiac failure
- flattening and sclerosis of the femoral or humeral heads secondary to AVN
- gallstones
- a small calcified spleen.

If a plain film demonstrating diffuse osteosclerosis is presented to a junior radiology trainee during a "hot seat" tutorial, they will undoubtedly blurt out fluorosis as the first diagnosis in their differential list of one . . . we have all seen or done this; however, this habit needs to be kicked, and now! Fluorosis is an extremely rare condition and has not made it into our mnemonic for that reason. Unless you see the obvious and characteristic ligamentous calcification of fluorosis, this diagnosis should be mentioned with caution in the exam, and then only at the end of your list of differential diagnoses. Examiners are more likely to appreciate a discussion of the more common conditions, such as renal osteodystrophy, metastatic disease, sickle cell disease and myelofibrosis.

Pearls

- List the more common differential diagnoses first: renal osteodystrophy, diffuse metastases, sickle cell disease and myelofibrosis.
- If the film is a CXR, look at the lateral clavicles for bone resorption. If present, consider renal osteodystrophy.
- Check for breast asymmetry on a CXR. If present, think about sclerotic metastases and look for axillary clips, lung nodules and lymphangitis.
- Metastatic disease is commonly secondary to breast cancer in females and prostate cancer in males.
- If the bones are strikingly and uniformly dense, consider congenital causes such as osteopetrosis and pyknodysostosis. These have associated bone fragility, so look for deformities that indicate previous pathological fracture.
- The paediatric conditions on this list can be differentiated using a lateral film of the skull and mandible. A normal size sclerotic mandible with supernumerary teeth is present in osteopetrosis, while a hypoplastic sclerotic mandible associated with multiple wormian bones is present in pyknodysostosis.
- If there are no obvious clues as to the likely diagnosis, mention that you have

searched for important discriminators such as evidence of malignancy, osteolysis and vertebral abnormalities.

- Avoid mentioning fluorosis unless you see convincing ligamentous calcification.

17.
Multiple lucent bone lesions

"Metastases May Eventually Fracture Bones"

	Condition	Associated features
M	Metastases	Generally occurs in those aged >40 years old Variable appearances Well or ill-defined but look for aggressive features Non-expansile or expansile May have a sclerotic component
M	Myeloma	Occurs in those aged >35 years old Well-defined lytic lesions of uniform size Endosteal scalloping (non-specific) Rarely sclerotic
E	Enchondromatosis (Ollier's disease/ Mafucci's syndrome)	Present in childhood Commonly in hands and wrists Multiple lytic, expansile, metaphyseal lesions Chondroid matrix (punctate/curvilinear foci of calcification within lesion) Abnormal growth, shortening and deformity of affected limbs Ollier's disease: many enchondromata Mafucci's syndrome: many enchondromata associated with soft tissue haemangiomas (phleboliths seen on plain film)
F	Fibrous dysplasia	Occurs in those aged <30 years old Especially ribs, pelvis and proximal femur, humerus, skull and mandible Diaphyseal or metaphyseal Usually well defined Endosteal scalloping Hazy, ground-glass internal matrix Thick sclerotic rim ("rind" sign) "Shepherd's crook" deformity – bowed proximal femur
B	Brown tumours	Variable appearance Well defined with some expansion Secondary features of hyperparathyroidism, e.g. subperiosteal bone resorption, "rugger jersey" spine, acro-osteolysis, osteopenia

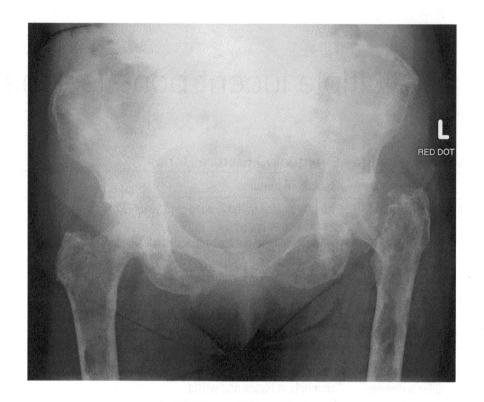

Diagnosis: Multiple myeloma

MODEL ANSWER

This is a frontal radiograph of the pelvis of an adult. There are multiple, well-circumscribed, lucent lesions within both proximal femora and the pubic rami. Some of these lesions demonstrate endosteal scalloping. There is a transcervical fracture of the left femoral neck, which is presumably pathological. There is no evidence of significant bony expansion, calcified internal matrix or periosteal reaction.

In summary, there are multiple lucent bony lesions. In an adult patient, the most likely diagnoses are metastatic disease or multiple myeloma. Brown tumours could also be considered, especially if there was any evidence of hyperparathyroidism.

To take this further, I would review the previous imaging and clinical history for evidence of known primary malignancy. If available, hand radiographs could be assessed for evidence of hyperparathyroidism. Serum and urine electrophoresis would identify paraproteins in keeping with myeloma. Raised calcium and parathyroid hormone levels would suggest hyperparathyroidism and brown tumours. If these tests were negative and no primary malignancy had been noted previously, I would organise a staging CT scan of the chest, abdomen and pelvis.

Discussion

There is significant overlap in the appearances of the conditions described here. However, metastases and myeloma are at the top of the list in the adult patient. It is essential to mention these two possible causes in both a viva and long case exam setting. Although less likely, brown tumours have a similar appearance, so it is good practice to look actively for the secondary signs of hyperparathyroidism – you may be shown a hand radiograph as a follow-on film.

As well as presenting with diffuse skeletal involvement, as in this case, myeloma may present as a single lesion (plasmacytoma), diffuse skeletal osteopenia (especially seen in the spine, where it often presents with multiple wedge compression fractures) and, rarely, sclerotic bony lesions.

It is difficult to distinguish between lytic metastases and myeloma on plain radiographs alone. Other modalities are helpful. The presence of a primary malignancy and other metastases on CT suggests metastatic disease. A bone scan may be abnormal in metastatic disease but will be normal in cases of myeloma, which is assessed with a series of plain radiographs known as a "skeletal survey". Non-radiological tests can also be recommended in your management plan – for example, urine and serum electrophoresis to look for the presence of monoclonal protein, as this is one of the diagnostic criteria for myeloma.

Fibrous dysplasia is usually diagnosed in childhood. Fibrous tissue forms in the medulla replacing the normal trabeculae and creating a lucent lesion. The fibrous tissue gradually calcifies and develops a ground-glass appearance, progressing to a sclerotic rim ("rind" sign) with eventual sclerosis and resolution. These lesions may be solitary (monostotic) or multiple (polyostotic). McCune–Albright's syndrome occurs in females and associates polyostotic fibrous dysplasia with precocious puberty and café-au-lait skin pigmentation.

Pearls

- Metastases and myeloma are at the top of the list of differential diagnoses in an adult patient and have a similar appearance on plain radiographs.
- Also mention brown tumours when presented with multiple lucent bone lesions.
- For further management, staging CT and isotope bone scans are reasonable imaging investigations; serum and protein electrophoresis as well as tests of calcium and parathyroid hormone (PTH) levels are good non-radiological investigations.

18.
Expansile lytic bone lesion

"Politicians Always Make Grave Blunders"

	Condition	Associated features
P	Plasmacytoma/ large myeloma deposit	Occurs in those aged >35 years old Well defined Any location May be multiple lesions if multiple myeloma
A	Aneurysmal bone cyst (ABC)	Occurs in those aged <30 years old Most common in long bones around the knee, proximal femur and spine Metaphyseal Well defined
M	Metastases	Occurs in those aged >40 years old Well or ill-defined, but look for aggressive features May be multiple Any location
G	Giant cell tumour (GCT)	Closed epiphysis Well-defined non-sclerotic margin Eccentric position Epiphyseal – the lesion must abut the articular surface Most commonly adjacent to the knee, the distal radius and sacrum
B	Brown tumours	Well defined Any location Look for evidence of hyperparathyroidism, e.g. subperiosteal bone resorption, osteosclerosis, soft tissue calcification

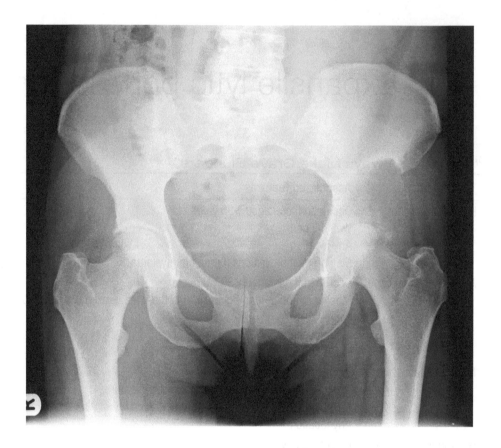

Diagnosis: Metastatic thyroid carcinoma

MODEL ANSWER

This is an AP radiograph of an adult pelvis and proximal femora. There is a solitary lucent and expansile lesion within the left ilium involving the left acetabulum. This has an ill-defined margin medially and a more well-defined margin superiorly. There is destruction of the lateral cortex of the ilium and the superior margin of the acetabulum.

In summary, there is an aggressive expansile lytic lesion within the left hemipelvis. This is most likely to represent a metastatic deposit. A plasmacytoma could also be considered. A primary bone tumour is much less likely. Thyroid and renal carcinomas are common causes of expansile lytic metastases; however, breast and lung metastases are also possible.

I would review the clinical history. In the absence of a known primary malignancy, I would discuss the case with the referring clinician and arrange a staging CT scan of the chest, abdomen and pelvis.

Discussion

There are several important features to mention when describing a bone lesion:
- whether it is solitary or there are multiple lesions
- its composition – lucent, sclerotic or mixed
- its position within the bone (epiphyseal, metaphyseal, diaphyseal)
- its position within the bone (cortical, medullary, central, eccentric etc.)
- its zone of transition – whether the margin is well or ill-defined
- whether it is expansile
- whether there is a periosteal reaction or not; if there is, whether it is benign or aggressive
- any additional features (fractures, cortical breach etc.).

In general, age is a useful discriminator when forming a diagnosis of a bone lesion. You will not be given the age of the patient in the exam and you should not need to ask for it. You can demonstrate your knowledge by describing the age of the patient in your first sentence using a term such as "adult", "child" or "infant". Signs of degenerative joint disease are more likely to be present in older adults rather than in someone in their twenties or thirties. You can also describe the skeleton as "fused" or "unfused" to signify age, although this is less specific.

Radiologists often use the terms "lucent" and "lytic" interchangeably. However, as the definition of "lysis" is a destructive process, the term "lucent" is more appropriate in an exam situation unless there is unequivocal evidence of bone destruction.

In this case, the margin of the lytic lesion has both well and ill-defined components. The presence of an ill-defined margin (or, to put it another way, a wide zone of transition), whether complete or not, suggests an aggressive process such as metastatic disease.

Pearls

- Always decide whether a lesion is aggressive or non-aggressive – make this the first statement in your summary.
- The main feature determining whether a lucent lesion is aggressive is its margin or zone of transition – always comment on this.
- Refer to a lesion as being "lytic" if there is convincing aggressive destruction of bone; otherwise, use the word "lucent".
- If a lesion is ill-defined and expansile, think metastases.
- Unfortunately, metastases can be well defined with a narrow zone of transition, but this is less likely.
- Expansile lytic metastases are classically thyroid or renal in origin.
- It is normal practice to obtain a staging CT of the chest, abdomen and pelvis with a new aggressive bone lesion to identify a primary cause.

19

Aggressive lytic lesion in a child

"LOSE ME"

	Condition	Associated features
L	Leukaemia	Variable appearance: • metaphyseal lucent lines • osteopenia • periosteal reaction • focal ill-defined lytic lesions • elevated erythrocyte sedimentation rate (ESR) and anaemia
O	Osteomyelitis	Variable appearance: • often metaphyseal • may have lucency, sclerosis, periosteal reaction and soft tissue mass
S	Sarcoma (osteogenic)	Generally occurs in those aged 10–20 years old Metaphyseal Lysis and sclerosis Aggressive periosteal reaction Soft tissue mass
E	Eosinophilic granuloma	Generally occurs in those aged <10 years old Usually diaphyseal Well or ill-defined Periosteal reaction possible
M	Metastasis (neuroblastoma)	Generally occurs in those aged <2 years old Ill-defined lytic lesions May be multiple Evidence of primary tumour on cross-sectional imaging
E	Ewing's sarcoma	Generally occurs in those aged 10–20 years old Diaphyseal Ill-defined lysis, may be permeative Sclerosis less common Aggressive periosteal reaction Soft tissue mass

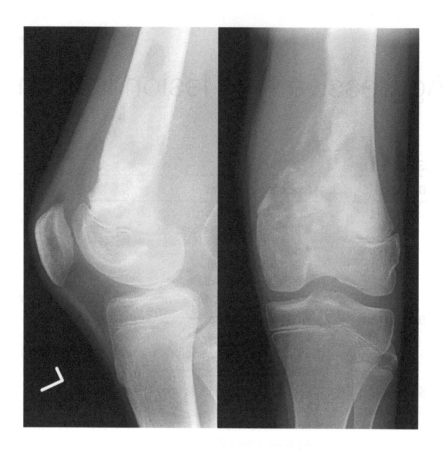

Diagnosis: Osteosarcoma

MODEL ANSWER

These are AP and lateral radiographs of the left knee of a child of school age. There is an aggressive lesion within the metaphysis of the left distal femur. The margins of the lesion are poorly defined with a wide zone of transition. The lesion has a mixed lytic and sclerotic pattern. There is cortical destruction of the posteromedial cortex and an associated aggressive periosteal reaction with a large soft tissue mass. There is cortical thinning and osteopenia of the proximal tibia in keeping with disuse osteoporosis.

In summary, there is an aggressive mixed lytic and sclerotic lesion within the left distal femoral metaphysis. This most likely represents an osteosarcoma. The differential diagnoses include Ewing's sarcoma, osteomyelitis and eosinophilic granuloma, but these are less likely.

To take this further, I would perform an MRI of the left distal femur using axial and coronal T1 and T2 fatsat [fat saturation] sequences to characterise the lesion, and large field of view T1 and STIR [short tau inversion recovery] sequences from the hip to the ankle to look for distant disease. I would also organise a bone scan and CT scan of the chest to assess for metastatic disease. An urgent referral to the regional bone tumour unit should be organised, for MDT discussion.

Discussion

It is important to establish whether a bone lesion is aggressive or non-aggressive on a plain radiograph, as this determines subsequent management. Two key features that indicate the rate of growth of a lesion – and therefore how aggressive it is likely to be – are the margins of the lesion and the nature of any periosteal reaction.

A bone lesion with a well-defined margin (narrow zone of transition) is a slow-growing lesion, and therefore non-aggressive. A lesion that is ill-defined (wide zone of transition), "moth-eaten" or permeative is a rapidly growing lesion, and therefore aggressive.

A smooth and solid periosteal reaction indicates that the insult to the cortical bone is progressing slowly and a non-aggressive process. The classic causes are osteoid osteoma, healing stress fracture and osteomyelitis. If the periosteum is elevated from the cortical bone (Codman's triangle), lamellated or spiculated (termed "sunburst"), this indicates an underlying aggressive process, such as bone sarcoma.

It is vital to realise that an aggressive periosteal reaction is not synonymous with an underlying malignancy. Osteomyelitis and eosinophilic granuloma can both produce an aggressive periosteal reaction. Therefore, in the exam setting, it is useful to describe bone lesions as being "aggressive" or "non-aggressive" rather than "benign" or "malignant".

It is difficult to differentiate between osteosarcoma and Ewing's sarcoma. Osteosarcoma is more commonly metaphyseal with some sclerosis. Ewing's sarcoma is commonly diaphyseal with permeative lysis. Unfortunately, these features can overlap.

The age of the patient narrows the list of differential diagnoses. Primary bone sarcoma is most commonly seen between 10 and 20 years of age. If the child is less than 5 years old, metastatic neuroblastoma and eosinophilic granuloma are more likely.

Pearls

- Look at the margin/zone of transition – is it well defined/narrow or ill-defined/wide?
- If the margin of a lesion demonstrates both well and ill-defined regions, the more aggressive pattern is the one that you should use to characterise the lesion.
- Characterise the periosteal reaction, if present – is it aggressive?
- After assessing the above features, decide if the lesion is aggressive or non-aggressive.
- Try to establish patient age by inspecting bone size and growth plates – in a toddler or infant, a primary bone sarcoma is less likely.
- Eosinophilic granuloma and osteomyelitis can mimic any aggressive bone lesion in a child and should be mentioned in the differential diagnoses.
- MRI is necessary for assessment of the soft tissues.
- The management plan for a suspected sarcoma should include a CT scan of the chest to assess for lung metastases and a bone scan to assess for skip lesions.

20

Epiphyseal lucent lesion in the young

"ACE GIG"

	Condition	Associated findings
A	ABC	Occurs in those aged 10–30 years old
		Epiphyseal and metaphyseal in the fused skeleton
		Most commonly metaphyseal in the unfused skeleton
		Well defined
		Expansile
		Cortical thinning
		Fluid–fluid levels (MRI)
		Also occurs in vertebral posterior elements
C	Chondroblastoma	Occurs in those aged 10–20 years old
		Eccentric epiphyseal lesion prior to skeletal fusion
		May extend into metaphysis after fusion
		Well defined
		Sclerotic margin
		Internal calcifications
		Florid bone marrow oedema (MRI)
E	Eosinophilic granuloma	Occurs in those aged <30 years old
		Variable appearance
		More often diaphyseal/metaphyseal than epiphyseal
		Well or ill-defined
		Lytic or sclerotic
		Periosteal reaction
G	GCT	Occurs in those aged 20–40 years old
		Fused growth plates
		Epiphyseal lesion expanding into the metaphysis
		Must abut the articular surface
		Eccentrically positioned lesion
		Well-defined non-sclerotic margin
		Expansile with cortical thinning
		No marrow oedema on MRI

	Condition	Associated findings
I	Infection	Occurs at any age
		Variable appearance
		Cortical sclerosis/breach
		Soft tissue swelling
		Periosteal reaction
		Sequestrum
		"Penumbra" sign on T1-weighted MRI
G	Geode	Less likely in a young patient
		Background of degenerative joint disease

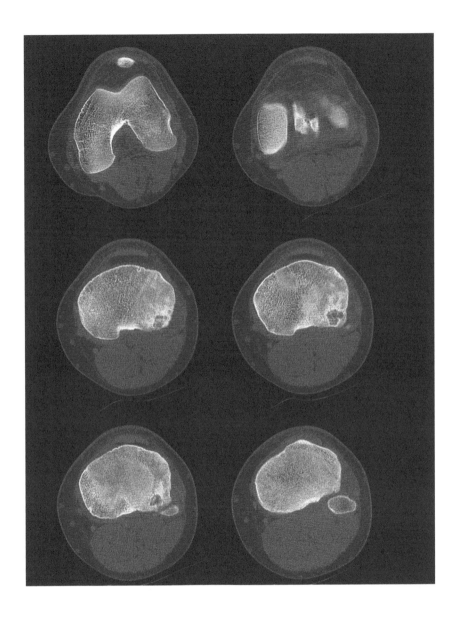

Diagnosis: Chondroblastoma

MODEL ANSWER

These are selected axial CT images of the knee joint and proximal tibia and fibula in a young patient. There is a well-defined, non-expansile, lucent lesion within the posterior tibial epiphysis. The lesion contains scattered foci of internal calcification and there is bony sclerosis of the margin. There is no periosteal reaction, cortical breach or endosteal scalloping.

In summary, there is a small, non-aggressive, lucent lesion within the proximal tibial epiphysis. The most likely diagnosis is a chondroblastoma. Osteomyelitis and giant cell tumour are possible differential diagnoses.

To take this further, I would review any previous plain radiographs and recent blood results. I would organise an MRI scan for further evaluation of the bone marrow and surrounding soft tissues. I would seek an urgent opinion from the local bone tumour unit.

(Images from an MRI scan are shown.)

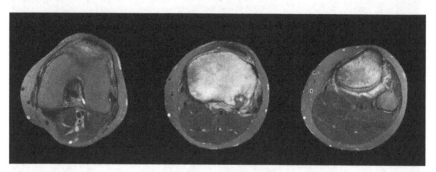

These are selected axial T2 fatsat images of the proximal tibia in the same patient. The previously described lesion demonstrates high signal centrally and low signal at its margin, in keeping with the sclerotic rim. There is a large area of high signal in the surrounding bone and soft tissues, in keeping with marked perilesional oedema. These features are in keeping with a chondroblastoma.

Discussion

It is very likely you will encounter a bone lesion during the viva part of the examination. There are simple strategies for approaching a bone lesion on any radiograph, CT or MRI scan. The main factors to consider are the patient's age (check whether the growth plates are fused or unfused), the location of the lesion (whether it is in the epiphysis, metaphysis or diaphysis; whether it is medullary or cortical) and the presence or absence of aggressive features (whether it is well or ill-defined, what type of periosteal reaction is evident, if there is a cortical breach). Try to verbalise your thought processes by describing each of these features in turn. These will narrow your list of differential diagnoses.

Some bone lesions have a classic appearance that leaves little doubt as to the diagnosis – such as a "fallen fragment" sign within a lucent lesion in a child's proximal humerus. In this situation you should not offer a list of differential diagnoses but confidently state your diagnosis to end the case. To be able to do this, it is essential you know the typical appearance and location of such classic lesions. These include simple bone cysts, fibrous dysplasia, osteosarcoma, enchondromatosis (Ollier's disease and Mafucci's syndrome) and multiple hereditary exostoses (also known as diaphyseal aclasis).

There are frequently cases, like the one described here, for which there are several sensible diagnostic possibilities, and in this situation a short (three is a good number to aim for) differential list of diagnoses should be offered. The epiphyseal location narrows the list to the conditions described in the table, and the three most likely in a young patient are chondroblastoma, GCT and osteomyelitis. The presence of surrounding sclerosis and lack of expansion goes against it being a GCT. Osteomyelitis remains a possibility, but the internal matrix goes against this.

Osteomyelitis can be difficult to distinguish from bone tumours. The presence of elevated inflammatory markers is more likely in, but not exclusive to, osteomyelitis. On T1-weighted MRI, the "penumbra" sign is suggestive of subacute osteomyelitis. This appears as a rim of T1 signal that is higher than that of the cavity it surrounds and is due to the vascular granulation tissue that surrounds an intraosseous abscess. The rim also enhances with contrast, which is not a feature of bone tumours.

A chondroblastoma is a rare benign bone tumour. It is the most common epiphyseal tumour in skeletally immature patients. It is usually seen in the long bones, especially around the knee but also in the apophyses (ossification centres that do not contribute to bone length), such as the patella and greater trochanter. There is some overlap with the imaging appearances of the other listed differential diagnoses, but a sclerotic rim, internal calcifications, florid surrounding marrow oedema and confinement to the epiphysis in an unfused skeleton support the diagnosis of chondroblastoma.

Pearls

- The top three differential diagnoses in a young patient with an epiphyseal lucent lesion are chondroblastoma, GCT and infection.
- Consider chondroblastoma when presented with an epiphyseal lesion that has a sclerotic rim with marked perilesional marrow oedema on MRI.
- Chondroblastoma is the commonest tumour of the patella.
- Always state whether the lesion appears non-aggressive or aggressive in your summary.
- "Lytic" means destructive, therefore aggressive. "Lucent" is a better term to use when describing a non-aggressive bone lesion.
- Above the age of 40 years, add metastases/myeloma and remove chondroblastoma from the list of differential diagnoses.
- MRI is usually sensible to assess the marrow and soft tissues.

21.
Diffuse bone marrow infiltration on magnetic resonance imaging

"MLML" or "Multiple Lytic Marrow Lesions"

	Condition	Associated features
M	Metastases Myeloma	Metastases: • more commonly focal rather than diffuse marrow involvement • usually low T1 and high T2/STIR signal. Sclerotic metastases are low signal on T1 and T2 sequences • may be evidence of a primary tumour – always check the localiser images Myeloma: • more commonly diffuse than focal • variable T2 signal – high or low
L	Lymphoma	Marrow appearance as for metastases More commonly focal than diffuse Usually secondary to extraosseous disease: lymphadenopathy, splenomegaly
M	Myelofibrosis Mastocytosis	Diffuse abnormality Splenomegaly – may be best seen on localiser images Very low T1 (black marrow) signal Low T2 signal
L	Leukaemia	Diffuse bone marrow abnormality Variable T2 signal

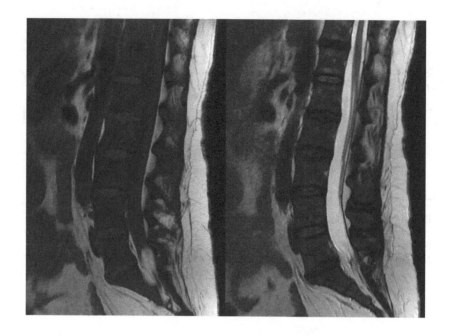

Diagnosis: Myelofibrosis

MODEL ANSWER

These are selected sagittal T1- and T2-weighted images of the lumbar spine in an adult. There is diffusely low T1 signal throughout the imaged bone marrow, which is of lower signal intensity than that of the intervertebral discs. There is heterogeneous low marrow signal throughout the lumbar spine and sacrum on the T2 fatsat images.

There is normal sagittal alignment of the lumbar spine. There is mild wedging of the L2 and L3 superior end plates but no central canal stenosis. Normal appearances of the conus and cauda equina. No significant extraosseous abnormality is demonstrated on the available images.

In summary, there is diffuse bone marrow infiltration. The differential diagnoses for this include myeloma, metastases, myelofibrosis, leukaemia and lymphoma.

To take this further, I would like to know if there is a history of lymphoma or malignancy. I would also like to review the localiser images for evidence of a primary tumour or splenomegaly. Appropriate investigations would include serum and urine electrophoresis and bone marrow aspirate. A staging CT scan and bone biopsy could also be considered.

(A coronal localiser image is then shown.)

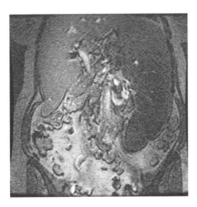

There is marked splenomegaly. The presence of diffuse marrow infiltration with splenomegaly is in keeping with a diagnosis of myelofibrosis.

Discussion

Normal bone marrow in the spine is of noticeably higher T1 signal intensity than the adjacent normal intervertebral discs. Diffuse marrow infiltration is characterised by a global reduction in T1 signal, similar to or lower than that of the normal intervertebral discs and muscle. This can be easily overlooked. However, most marrow pathology is also of high signal on T2 fatsat and STIR sequences.

The appearance of diffuse very low T1 signal (black marrow) with a corresponding low T2 signal in the vertebrae raises the possibility of sclerotic metastases (e.g. breast and prostate), mastocytosis, myelofibrosis and osteopetrosis.

MRI can identify diffuse marrow infiltration but cannot easily establish a cause. Further investigations are required to establish a diagnosis, as described.

Pearls

- On T1-weighted images, the marrow is abnormal if it has a signal that is the same or darker than that of the intervertebral discs.
- Diffuse marrow infiltration on MRI is a non-specific finding.
- Look for abnormalities outside the spine to suggest a diagnosis, such as retroperitoneal nodes, splenomegaly or lung and renal masses. The localiser images are particularly useful for this.
- Metastases and lymphoma more commonly produce focal rather than diffuse marrow abnormalities.

22.
Posterior vertebral body scalloping

"SALMON"

	Condition	Associated features
S	Spinal cord tumour	Localised widening of the interpedicular distance at tumour site
A	Achondroplasia Acromegaly	Achondroplasia: • short pedicles resulting in sagittal spinal canal narrowing • progressive caudal narrowing of interpedicular distance • anterior vertebral body beaks • "champagne glass" pelvic inlet • horizontal sacrum • "tombstone" iliac wings Acromegaly: enlarged vertebral bodies in both AP and lateral dimensions
M	Marfan's syndrome Morquio's syndrome	Marfan's syndrome: • scoliosis • pectus excavatum/carinatum Morquio's syndrome: • platyspondyly/vertebra plana • central anterior vertebral body beaks • hypoplastic dens • atlanto-axial instability
O	Osteogenesis imperfecta	Osteopenia with multiple vertebral wedge fractures, resulting in biconcave vertebral bodies
N	NF-1	Thoracolumbar kyphoscoliosis Absent or eroded pedicles Expansion of the intervertebral foramina due to "dumbbell" neurofibromas Hypoplastic vertebrae

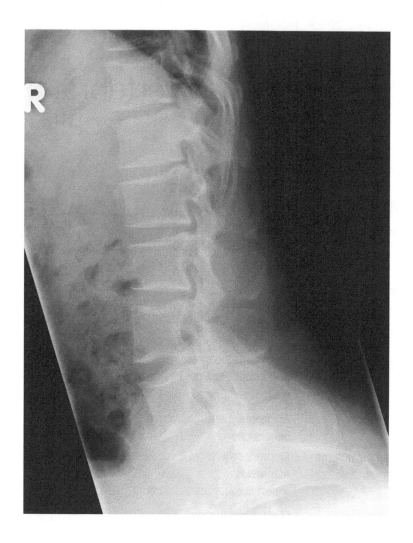

Diagnosis: Achondroplasia

Definition: An abnormal increased concavity of the posterior cortex of the vertebral body. This may occur in one or more vertebral bodies and is most commonly seen in the lumbar spine. It is best demonstrated on the lateral radiograph, sagittal CT images and by MRI.

MODEL ANSWER

This is a plain lateral radiograph of the lumbar spine in an adult patient. There is an exaggerated concavity of the posterior cortex of multiple lumbar vertebral bodies, most markedly at L4 and L5. The pedicles are truncated and the spinal canal is narrowed. The vertebral body heights are reasonably well maintained. There are no destructive bone lesions. The bone density appears normal. I note that the sacrum has a horizontal orientation.

In summary, there is posterior vertebral body scalloping associated with a horizontal sacrum and shortened pedicles. These findings are in keeping with achondroplasia.

To take this further, I would like to review an AP radiograph of the lumbar spine and pelvis to look for progressive caudal narrowing of the interpedicular distances, "tombstone" iliac wings and a "champagne-glass" pelvic inlet.

(If the examiner remains silent at this point, they are inviting you to continue . . .)

The differential diagnoses for posterior vertebral body scalloping also include a spinal cord tumour, acromegaly, Marfan's syndrome, mucopolysaccharidoses (such as Morquio's syndrome), osteogenesis imperfecta and neurofibromatosis.

In the absence of a known associated musculoskeletal condition, an MRI of the spine would be useful to assess for a tumour within the spinal canal and dural ectasia.

Discussion

The diagnoses for posterior vertebral body scalloping can be grouped into three categories, by aetiology:

1. increased pressure within the spinal canal due to a slow-growing mass, such as an ependymoma
2. dural ectasia, which is the ballooning of the dural sac due to an underlying weakness of the dura. This is a feature of connective tissue diseases and is seen in Marfan's syndrome, neurofibromatosis and osteogenesis imperfecta
3. congenital skeletal conditions such as achondroplasia and Morquio's syndrome.

Pearls

- It is unlikely that you will be able to distinguish between these different conditions on a single lateral radiograph without secondary features.
- Look for short pedicles; spinal canal narrowing; horizontal sacrum (achondroplasia); platyspondyly (Morquio's syndrome); widened intervertebral foramina, focal vertebral erosions or hypoplasia (neurofibromatosis); wedge fractures or osteopenia (osteogenesis imperfecta); and anterior vertebral body beaking.
- If there are no obvious secondary features of the lateral lumbar spine film, useful further investigations to ask for would include an AP view of the lumbar spine to assess the pedicle widths, an AP view of the pelvis to look for any evidence of achondroplasia and an MRI of the lumbar spine to look for dural ectasia or a mass within the spinal canal. If you suspect acromegaly, a hand radiograph may allow you to confirm this by showing the characteristic signs.
- In an exam situation, the probable causes of posterior vertebral scalloping are achondroplasia, Marfan's syndrome and neurofibromatosis, as these are multisystem disorders. Learn the various manifestations of these conditions as these are likely to form the basis of your dialogue with the examiner.

23.
Lateral clavicle resorption

"SHIRT"

	Condition	Associated features
S	Scleroderma	Dilated oesophagus
		Lower lobe fibrosis
		Soft tissue calcification
H	Hyperparathyroidism	Osteosclerosis
		Other areas of osteolysis
		Brown tumours
		Soft tissue calcification
I	Infection (osteomyelitis)	Unilateral
R	RA	Glenohumeral erosions and joint space narrowing
		Loss of the subacromial space
		Lower lobe fibrosis
		Signs of AVN due to steroid use, e.g. humeral head sclerosis
T	Trauma (post-traumatic osteolysis)	Old fracture
		Unilateral

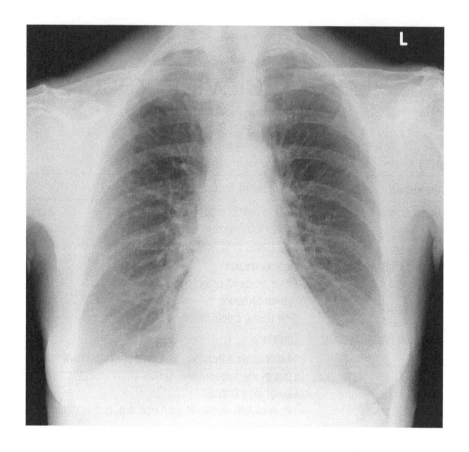

Diagnosis: RA

MODEL ANSWER

This is a frontal chest radiograph of an adult female. There is extensive bone resorption of the lateral ends of both clavicles. No other areas of bone resorption or other bony abnormality are visible. There is loss of the left subacromial space, likely due to degenerative changes of the rotator cuff. No obvious erosive changes can be seen in the humeral heads.

The lungs are clear with no evidence of lower lobe fibrosis. The cardiomediastinal contour is normal. The oesophagus is not dilated. The soft tissues are normal.

In summary, there is bilateral resorption of the lateral clavicles. This is most likely due to a systemic disorder such as hyperparathyroidism, rheumatoid arthritis or scleroderma.

To take this further, I would review any previous imaging – in particular, a radiograph of the hands – to assess for the presence of an erosive arthropathy, phalangeal resorption, soft tissue calcification or acro-osteolysis.

Discussion

Hyperparathyroidism is the uncontrolled excess production of PTH.

Primary hyperparathyroidism is due to one or more hyperfunctioning parathyroid glands. This is most commonly due to a parathyroid adenoma, with parathyroid hyperplasia and carcinoma being much rarer causes.

Secondary hyperparathyroidism occurs in response to low calcium levels. It results in compensatory hyperplasia of all four parathyroid glands. The most common cause of secondary hyperparathyroidism is chronic renal failure.

There are multiple typical radiological features of hyperparathyroidism:
- bone resorption – especially of the distal phalanges (acro-osteolysis) and radial margins of the middle phalanges. Also the ribs, humeri and femora
- brown tumours: lytic bone lesions, often expansile and multiple
- osteosclerosis and "rugger jersey" spine – more common in secondary hyperparathyroidism
- soft tissue calcification – more common in secondary hyperparathyroidism
- chondrocalcinosis, the deposition of calcium pyrophosphate in articular tissues – more common in primary hyperparathyroidism
- periostitis
- nephrocalcinosis
- bone scan – a "superscan" can be seen in secondary but not primary hyperparathyroidism.

Scleroderma, also known as systemic sclerosis, is a multisystem connective tissue disorder. The main radiological features are:
- lower zone interstitial fibrosis (pleural disease is uncommon)
- oesophageal dilatation
- small bowel dilatation with crowding of valvulae conniventes – "stack of coins" appearance on barium studies
- acro-osteolysis with associated atrophy and tightening of the overlying soft tissues
- subcutaneous and periarticular calcification – calcinosis circumscripta
- sometimes superior rib notching.

RA is characterised by a symmetrical, deforming, proximal, erosive arthropathy that typically affects multiple metacarpophalangeal joints of both hands. There may be associated periarticular osteoporosis. The thoracic manifestations, which are relatively common in advanced disease, include:
- lower zone interstitial fibrosis
- rheumatoid nodules, which may cavitate but do not calcify
- pleural thickening and effusion, which is usually unilateral
- erosive arthropathy of the glenohumeral joints
- loss of the subacromial space due to rotator cuff atrophy/tear
- sometimes superior rib notching.

The most likely causes of bilateral resorption of the lateral clavicle are the listed systemic disorders. Each condition has characteristic features, which may or may not be visible on the chest radiograph provided. A radiograph of the hands could help to distinguish between the three diagnoses.

Pearls

- Assess if the resorption is unilateral or bilateral: infection and post-traumatic osteolysis are likely to be unilateral, while connective tissue diseases and hyperparathyroidism are likely to be bilateral.
- Look for glenohumeral joint arthropathy (RA), lower lobe fibrosis (scleroderma or RA), dilated oesophagus (scleroderma) and any previous fracture (post-traumatic osteolysis).
- A radiograph of the hands will help narrow the list of differential diagnoses: ask for this.
- Be aware of the eponymous syndromes associated with RA, such as Caplan's and Felty's.

24.
Short metacarpals

"TIPS" or "The fingerTIPS are short"

	Condition(s)	Associated features
T	Turner's syndrome	Madelung's deformity
I	Idiopathic	Bony deformity
	Injury	Evidence of previous surgery
	Iatrogenic	
	Infection	
P	Pseudohypoparathyroidism	Intracranial calcification
	Pseudopseudohypoparathyroidism	(pseudohypoparathyroidism)
S	Sickle cell disease (post-dactylitis)	Bone infarcts
		Deformity

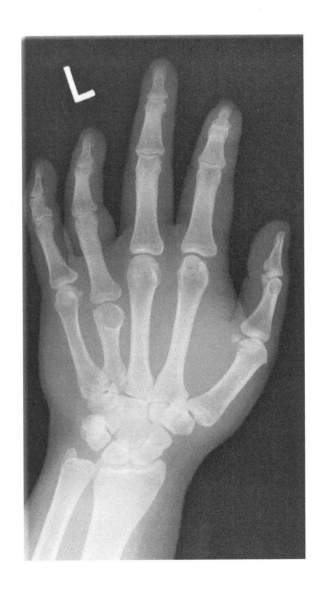

Diagnosis: Pseudohypoparathyroidism

MODEL ANSWER

This is an AP radiograph of the left hand of an adult patient. There is marked shortening of the fourth metacarpal. No associated Madelung's deformity is evident. The bones and joints otherwise appear normal. In particular, there is no bony deformity to suggest previous trauma, no evidence of previous surgery, focal bony lesions or soft tissue calcifications.

In summary, there is shortening of the left fourth metacarpal with no evidence of other bone or joint abnormality.

The most common cause of this abnormality is idiopathic; however, there are a number of conditions associated with short metacarpals. These include pseudohypoparathyroidism and pseudopseudohypoparathyroidism, previous trauma, surgery, infection and sickle cell dactylitis. In a female, I would also consider Turner's syndrome.

To take this further, I would review the patient history and examine any previous imaging. If the patient has had a CT scan of the head, the presence of intracranial calcification would be in keeping with a diagnosis of pseudohypoparathyroidism or pseudopseudohypoparathyroidism.

Discussion

Pseudohypoparathyroidism is an X-linked dominant condition in which there is end-organ resistance to PTH. PTH levels are elevated, but serum calcium levels remain low. It is associated with short fourth and fifth metacarpals and metatarsals. Intracranial and soft tissue calcifications may also be present. Other features include short stature.

Individuals with pseudopseudohypoparathyroidism have a similar phenotype to those with pseudohypoparathyroidism, but are biochemically normal.

Turner's syndrome is exclusively found in females (chromosomal pattern 45XO). In this condition, the fourth metacarpal is shortened, with or without shortening of the third and/or fifth metacarpals. There is an association between Turner's syndrome and Madelung's deformity. This is an important positive or negative finding when presented with an AP view of the hands with shortened metacarpals, and should be commented upon. Patients with Turner's syndrome commonly also have a cubitus valgus deformity. This condition is also associated with short stature, scoliosis and kyphosis, aortic coarctation, and horseshoe kidney. This multisystem condition may be well suited to a long case question.

Sickle cell disease can cause growth arrest, resulting in a shortened metacarpal. In such cases, there may be evidence of previous bone infarcts which could appear as focal areas of sclerotic bone and residual deformity. Infection may similarly impede bone growth.

Pearls

- Look for and comment upon Madelung's deformity of the distal radius: Turner's syndrome has an association with Madelung's deformity.
- Pseudohypoparathyroidism is end-organ resistance to PTH resulting in low serum calcium and high PTH; pseudopseudohypoparathyroidism has a similar phenotype but with normal biochemistry.

25.
Acro-osteolysis

"SPINACH"

	Condition	Associated features
S	Scleroderma	Soft tissue calcification Symmetrical erosive polyarthropathy Sclerodactyly – skin atrophy of the fingertips Flexion contractures of the fingers
P	Psoriasis	Symmetrical erosive distal arthropathy of the hands Periostitis/bone proliferation "Pencil-in-cup" deformity Psoriatic nail changes may be seen on film Bony ankylosis of distal interphalangeal/proximal interphalangeal (PIP) joints
I	Injury (e.g. burns, frostbite) Infection	
N	Neuropathy (e.g. diabetes, leprosy)	
C	Congenital (Hajdu–Cheney's syndrome)	
H	Hyperparathyroidism	Subperiosteal bone resorption, classically on radial aspect of the middle phalanges Brown tumours Osteosclerosis Dystrophic soft tissue calcification

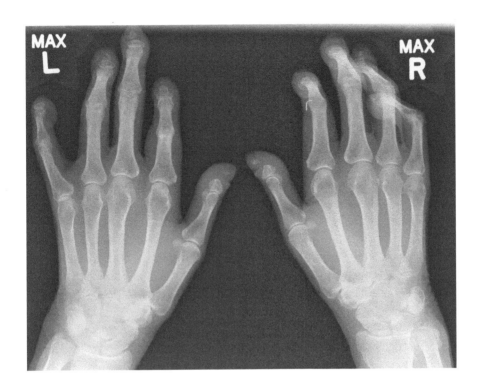

Diagnosis: Scleroderma

Definition: Bone resorption of the terminal aspect of the distal phalanges (usually multiple digits)

MODEL ANSWER

This is a radiograph of both hands of an adult patient. There is extensive bone resorption of the tufts of multiple distal phalanges bilaterally. The PIP joints of multiple digits are flexed, most prominently in the right hand, suggestive of contractures. There is no soft tissue calcification, periostitis or more proximal bone resorption. The bone density is normal.

In summary, there is acro-osteolysis affecting multiple digits of the hand with likely flexion contractures or sclerodactyly. The most likely diagnosis is scleroderma. Hyperparathyroidism is less likely due to the absence of middle phalangeal subperiosteal bone resorption. Psoriatic arthropathy is also less likely due to the absence of periostitis and new bone formation. If there is a relevant history, thermal injury and infection may also be considered.

To take this further, I would review the patient history and compare this radiograph with any previous imaging. A chest radiograph may show evidence of oesophageal dilatation or basal fibrotic change.

Discussion

It is important to mention pertinent negative findings on a viva film, as these can help narrow the list of differential diagnoses and demonstrate knowledge to the examiner, as seen in the model answer here.

Pearls

- Look for soft tissue calcification, sclerodactyly, new bone formation/periostitis and bony resorption of the radial aspect of the middle phalanges.
- Remember to mention previous thermal injury and infection as possible causes.
- If there is focal destruction of a single distal phalanx, consider a different set of diagnoses: metastasis (most likely due to lung carcinoma: check for HOA), dermoid cyst (which involves the palmar aspect), glomus tumour (which involves the dorsal aspect) and infection.

26.
Bowed tibia

"PROBING"

	Condition	Associated features
P	Paget's disease	Anterior bowing Cortical thickening Coarsened trabeculae Almost always involves the epiphyseal region "Banana" insufficiency fracture anteriorly Found in older people – rare in those <40 years of age
R	Rickets	Frayed, splayed and cupped metaphyses Widened growth plates
O	Osteogenesis imperfecta	Osteopenia Multiple fractures Involves whole skeleton
B	Blount's disease (tibia vara)	Depression and beaking of the proximal tibial metaphysis Medial deviation of the tibia distally
I	Idiopathic	
N	NF-1	Anterolateral tibial bowing, at the junction of the middle and distal third Fibular hypoplasia Pathological fracture Pseudoarthrosis Also associated with *many* other skeletal abnormalities, e.g. sphenoid wing dysplasia, lambdoidal suture defect, "ribbon" ribs, posterior vertebral scalloping, kyphoscoliosis
G	abnormal Growth, e.g. achondroplasia	Shortening of the long bones Flared metaphyses Typical spinal and pelvic features, e.g. posterior vertebral scalloping, decreased caudal interpedicular distance, "tombstone" iliac wings, horizontal sacrum

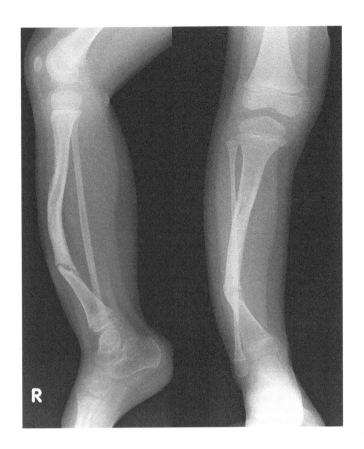

Diagnosis: NF-1

Definition: Abnormal curvature of the tibia

MODEL ANSWER

This is an AP and lateral radiograph of the right lower leg of a young child. There is marked anterolateral bowing of the right tibia. There is an ununited undisplaced fracture at the apex of the angulation, which lies at the junction of the middle and distal thirds of the tibia. There is some adjacent thickening and sclerosis of the tibial cortex. The fibula and distal femur have a normal appearance. No soft tissue nodules are demonstrated. There is normal bone density and no evidence of metaphyseal abnormality.

In summary, there is anterolateral bowing of the distal tibia with an associated fracture. The findings are most likely to represent a skeletal manifestation of neurofibromatosis. The normal metaphyses and bone density make osteogenesis imperfecta and rickets less likely.

To take this further, I would correlate these findings with the clinical history and review any previous imaging for features of neurofibromatosis, such as posterior vertebral scalloping, "ribbon" ribs and sphenoid wing dysplasia.

Discussion

The case shown demonstrates just one of the many skeletal manifestations of NF-1. The classical appearance in the tibia is of anterolateral bowing, sometimes with an associated fracture of the lower tibia (as in this case). If advanced, there may be a frank pseudoarthrosis ("false joint") with tapering and/or cupping of bone ends at the fracture site. It is worth checking the soft tissues for the subtle appearance of subcutaneous neurofibromas, which will support your diagnosis. Additional films may be shown illustrating further features of NF-1 in other parts of the body (some of which are listed), so you will need to be aware of these.

For the purposes of the exam, severe lower limb deformity is most probably due to NF-1 or osteogenesis imperfecta. Both may have marked bowing of the tibia and fibula with gracile bones and pseudoarthroses. However, in osteogenesis imperfecta, there is more likely to be:

- reduced bone density (osteopenia and thin cortices)
- sclerotic transverse lines in the long bones (resulting from bisphosphonate therapy)
- multiple fractures
- extensive callus formation
- distant secondary features of multiple wormian bones and platyspondyly.

Pearls

- Comment on the bone density, metaphyses and direction of bowing.
- Anterolateral bowing is typical of NF-1.
- The deformity is often severe in NF-1 and osteogenesis imperfecta. Bone density and evidence of previous fractures will help you to distinguish between them.
- Rickets, Blount's disease and achondroplasia have characteristic metaphyseal abnormalities.
- Anterior bowing is associated with syphilis as well as Paget's disease.

27.
Diffuse periosteal reaction in adults

"Healthy People Take Vitamins"

	Condition	Associated features
H	HOA (secondary)	Usually smooth, bilateral and symmetrical
		Diaphyseal and metaphyseal, sparing epiphyses
		Long bones, tubular bones of hands/feet
		Associated lytic bone lesions (metastases)
		Affects an older age group than pachydermoperiostosis
P	Pachydermoperiostosis (primary HOA)	Can affect epiphyses (at tendon insertions) and metaphyses
		Rare; much less common than secondary HOA
		Presents in children and young adults
T	Thyroid acropachy	Usually spiculated fluffy periostitis
		Asymmetrical distribution
		Hands and/or feet are involved, not long bones
		Soft tissue swelling
V	Venous insufficiency	Lower limb
		Thick undulating periosteal reaction
		Phleboliths
		Soft tissue defects/bandages due to ulcers

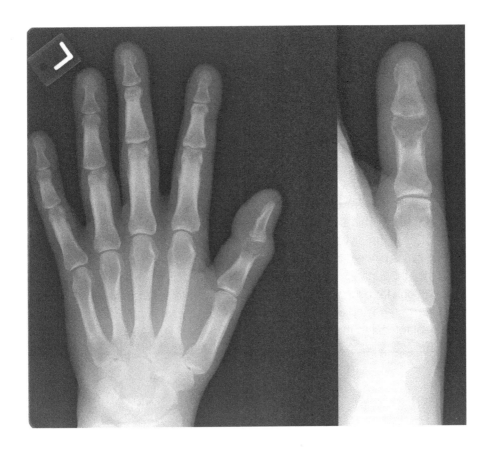

Diagnosis: HOA secondary to lung carcinoma

MODEL ANSWER

This is a radiograph of the left hand and a second view of the thumb in an adult. There is smooth uniform periosteal thickening along the metaphyses and diaphyses of multiple phalanges, most prominently along the thumb metacarpal and proximal phalanx. There is also a solitary ill-defined lytic lesion within the head of the proximal phalanx of the thumb. This lesion breaches the cortex and appears aggressive.

In summary, there is diffuse smooth periosteal reaction along multiple phalanges of the left hand. This is in keeping with hypertrophic osteoarthropathy. The presence of an aggressive lytic lesion in the thumb suggests that this is due to metastatic carcinoma of the lung.

To take this further, I would review the clinical history and recent imaging of the chest to look for a lung tumour. If this is an incidental finding, I would organise a chest radiograph and discuss these findings with the referring clinician to suggest an urgent referral to the chest physicians.

Discussion

HOA (secondary) is a paraneoplastic syndrome characterised by periosteal new bone formation, clubbing of the digits and arthritis. Radiographically, there is usually smooth and uniform periosteal new bone formation. This occurs within the diaphyses and metaphyses of distal long bones and sometimes the tubular bones of the hands and feet, as in this case. The clubbing of fingertips and soft tissue swelling are frequently seen but not specific to this condition.

Pachydermoperiostosis (primary HOA) is an autosomal dominant condition. It occurs in a younger age group than secondary HOA and has a slightly different distribution of periostitis, which begins in the epiphyses at tendon/ligament insertions. The epiphyses are usually spared in secondary HOA.

Secondary HOA is most commonly secondary to lung malignancy, but there are numerous causes, some of which are benign:

- lung: bronchogenic carcinoma (most common), abscess, bronchiectasis
- pleural: fibroma, mesothelioma
- cardiac: cyanotic heart disease
- abdominal: cirrhosis, inflammatory bowel disease.

In the stressful viva setting, diffuse periosteal thickening may not be immediately apparent. Therefore, when confronted with a plain radiograph for which you cannot easily spot the abnormality, train yourself to look at the periosteum (and, similarly, for radial resorption of the middle phalanges on a hand radiograph in hyperparathyroidism). A symmetrical smooth periosteal reaction is most likely to be due to HOA, which is most likely to be secondary to thoracic malignancy. Once you have spotted this abnormality, your reflex should be to ask for a CXR to look for a lung or pleural tumour.

Pearls

- Check for a subtle periosteal reaction when presented with a plain radiograph with no striking abnormality.
- Ask for a CXR when you have identified diffuse periosteal reaction.
- Look for non-specific findings such as clubbing, osteopenia and soft tissue swelling.
- Venous insufficiency is not a cause of periosteal reaction in the hands.
- Secondary HOA is much more common than primary HOA.
- The aetiology of secondary HOA may be divided into lung, pleural, cardiac and gastrointestinal causes.
- Metastases to the fingers and thumb are rare but most often caused by a primary lung carcinoma.

28.
Osteonecrosis of the hips (avascular necrosis)

"SAD GITS"

	Condition	Associated features
S	Steroids	Renal transplant
A	Alcohol	Pancreatic calcification (chronic pancreatitis)
D	Diabetes	Vascular calcification
G	Gaucher's disease	Massive splenomegaly
		Bone marrow infiltration
		Long bone abnormalities – Erlenmeyer flask, osteopenia, osteosclerosis
		Pathological fractures
		Multiple bone infarcts
		H-shaped vertebrae
I	Infection	Idiopathic: Perthes' disease in a child aged 4–8 years old –
	Inflammation	usually unilateral
	Idiopathic	
T	Trauma	Evidence of previous femoral neck fracture
S	Sickle cell anaemia	"Codfish"/H-shaped vertebrae
		Calcified/absent spleen
		Gallstones
		Bone infarcts
		Sclerotic bones

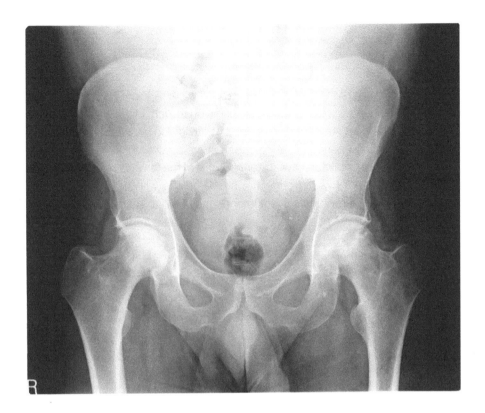

Diagnosis: Bilateral hip AVN secondary to steroid use

MODEL ANSWER

This is a plain radiograph of the pelvis of an adult patient. There is patchy sclerosis of both femoral heads, with a focal cystic lesion on the left. In the left femoral head, there is a subtle linear subchondral lucency. There is also possible flattening of the right femoral head superiorly. The joint spaces are preserved.

The findings are of bilateral avascular necrosis of the femoral heads. The cause is not demonstrated. I would correlate these findings with the patient's history. Assessment of any previous relevant images may help to define the chronicity.

An MRI scan would be useful to better define the extent of current marrow involvement.

(MR images are then shown.)

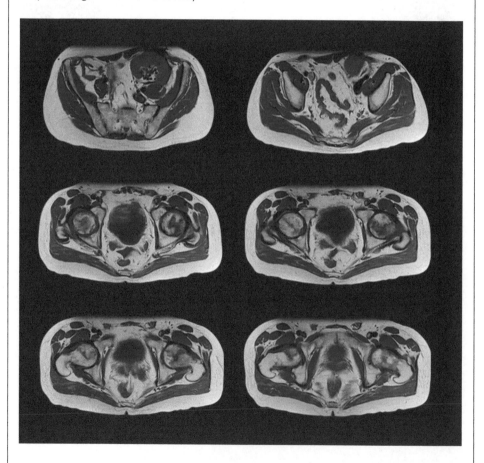

These are selected axial T1-weighted images through the pelvis of an adult patient.

There is a transplanted kidney in the left iliac fossa. There are serpentine low signal lines in both femoral heads and necks as well as scattered areas of low T1 signal.

The appearances are of bilateral osteonecrosis of the femoral heads. The renal transplant suggests that the cause is likely due to the use of steroids and other immunosuppressive drugs post-transplant.

To take this further, I would review any available T2 fatsat images to assess the extent of the corresponding bone marrow oedema.

Discussion

Osteonecrosis is synonymous with AVN and bone infarcts. The femoral head is the most common site. Traditionally, AVN refers to osteonecrosis involving the epiphysis of a bone, and bone infarct when the metaphysis or diaphysis is involved. There are many possible causes for this and the more common causes are mentioned here.

T1-weighted MRI is highly sensitive and specific for osteonecrosis. The typical T1 appearance of early osteonecrosis is of a low signal subcortical serpentine line. There is often a corresponding "double line" sign on T2-weighted imaging. This appears as a high signal line just inside the low signal subcortical serpentine line, but this feature is not required to make the diagnosis.

Plain radiographs of early femoral head osteonecrosis are often normal, but findings vary and can include focal osteopenia and osteosclerosis. In more advanced disease, an irregular bony contour and collapse of the femoral head can be seen. The classic plain film finding in osteonecrosis is a curvilinear subchondral lucent line in the femoral head. This is known as the "crescent" sign and indicates imminent bony collapse. This is a typical case in the rapid reporting section of the examination.

In the exam setting, you may be presented with a case that illustrates the typical features of osteonecrosis. However, there may well be an additional feature on the image that suggests the most likely cause. You should actively look for these secondary features and vocalise your thought process as you go, even if these findings are not present. This will impress the examiner and help you to work through the list of differential diagnoses. Possible secondary features include a renal transplant (as in this case) or H-shaped vertebrae with a calcified spleen. Another example is of bilateral hip AVN with a large soft tissue mass arising from the left upper quadrant, pointing you towards the diagnosis of Gaucher's disease with splenomegaly. Other associations are described earlier in the table.

Pearls

- Serpentine subcortical low signal lines on T1-weighted images are specific for osteonecrosis.
- In the presence of osteonecrosis of the femoral heads, the key review areas are the lumbar vertebra (look for abnormal endplates), the right upper quadrant (for gallstones) and left upper quadrant (check spleen size).
- On MRI, assess the rest of the imaged marrow for further abnormalities. These may demonstrate marrow infiltration, fractures or bone infarcts.
- When there are features of osteonecrosis on a background of multiple skeletal abnormalities, consider sickle cell anaemia and Gaucher's disease.

Section 3

Gastrointestinal and genitourinary

29.
Enhancing liver lesion

"Medical Families All Hate Hospitals"

	Condition	Associated features
M	Metastasis (hypervascular)	Peripheral ring enhancement in the arterial phase, most commonly Variable appearance
F	Focal nodular hyperplasia (FNH)	Stellate central scar with high T2 signal Intense homogeneous enhancement of the mass in the arterial phase Mass becomes isointense to normal liver parenchyma (equilibrates) in the delayed phases Enhancement of the central scar in the delayed phase only
A	Adenoma	Heterogeneous, with patchy high T1 signal (fat and acute haemorrhage) Homogeneous enhancement in the arterial phase Remains hyperintense to normal liver with heterogeneous enhancement in the more delayed phases May have an apparent capsule
H	Haemangioma	Very high T2 signal Peripheral nodular enhancement in the arterial phase Subsequent centripetal infilling of contrast in the more delayed phases No delayed phase contrast washout
H	HCC	Evidence of cirrhosis Homogeneous or heterogeneous arterial phase enhancement Rapid contrast washout (reduced enhancement on the more delayed phase images) May invade the portal vein – a tumour thrombus will enhance; a bland thrombus will not

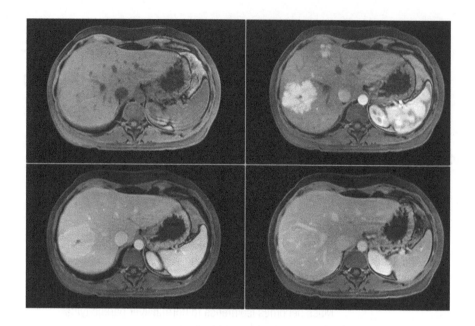

Diagnosis: FNH

MODEL ANSWER

These are selected T1-weighted images of the liver in an adult patient, acquired pre-contrast and post-contrast in the arterial, portal venous and equilibrium phases.

There are two lesions within the liver. These are both isointense to the surrounding liver parenchyma pre-contrast.

The larger lesion is within segments 7 and 8. In the arterial phase, it enhances avidly, but gradually becomes isointense to the normal liver in the delayed/equilibrium phase. This lesion has a central scar with enhancement in the delayed phase only.

There is a smaller lesion within segments 8 and 4a that exhibits a similar enhancement pattern. There is a central scar, but this is less obvious.

The liver has a smooth outline and is of normal size. The portal vein is patent.

In summary, there are two lesions in the right lobe of the liver that demonstrate the characteristic appearances of focal nodular hyperplasia. This is a benign lesion and does not require any follow-up.

Discussion

A typical FNH is an "Aunt Minnie" or "spot diagnosis" exam case, and therefore does not require a differential diagnosis. However, the examiner may go on to test your knowledge of the other enhancing liver lesions and how you would differentiate between them.

You should be able to recognise and name the different contrast phases used in a liver MRI from the images alone. This information will not usually be given to you directly. However, always quickly check the film details as occasionally the phase information may be recorded there. Spotting this will impress the examiner and will save you time and stress. The arterial phase is acquired 25–35 seconds after the administering intravenous contrast, and can be recognised because the contrast is very bright within the aorta. The portal venous phase is at 60–70 seconds, with the contrast now brightest within the portal veins. Delayed or equilibrium phases are acquired typically at 150, 300 and, very occasionally, 600 seconds. The contrast now appears generally less bright in all the vessels.

Arterial enhancement patterns are a good discriminator. Ring enhancement suggests a metastasis, a peripheral nodular pattern suggests a haemangioma, and a homogeneous pattern suggests an FNH or adenoma (an FNH may have a central scar and will equilibrate on delayed phases; an adenoma will be bright on T1 and will not equilibrate). In a cirrhotic liver, a lesion that shows arterial enhancement should make you consider an HCC.

The principle of washout is important. Eighty per cent of the blood supply to the liver parenchyma is supplied by the portal vein and 20% by the hepatic artery. Therefore, the liver enhances maximally in the portal venous phase. Most metastases are hypovascular, and most easily seen in the portal venous phase. Hypervascular metastases and HCCs gain their blood supply from the hepatic artery, thus enhance earlier than the normal liver parenchyma and demonstrate early contrast washout (becoming hypointense to the normal liver) in the portal venous and delayed phases.

Pearls

- Enhancing liver lesions are most easily differentiated on the arterial phase of a contrast study.
- A CT or MR scan in the arterial phase will show a very bright aorta due to the contrast within it.
- A typical FNH demonstrates avid arterial enhancement, becoming isointense to the liver on the portal venous phase. There may be a central scar with high T2 signal and delayed enhancement.
- Look at the liver size and contour. An arterially enhancing lesion with delayed phase washout in a cirrhotic liver is characteristic of an HCC.
- Most metastases are hypovascular and do not enhance in the arterial phase.

- Hypervascular metastases may be seen in renal and thyroid carcinoma as well as carcinoid, pancreatic islet cell tumours and melanoma.
- Try to use the segmental anatomy of the liver when describing liver lesions. If in doubt, stick to right and left lobes to avoid making a mistake.

30.
Air in the biliary tree (pneumobilia)

"Grovelling Surgeons Expect Immediate CT Scans"

	Condition	Associated features
G	Gallstone ileus	Small bowel dilatation/obstruction Gallstone within the terminal ileum
S	Surgery (biliary-enteric)	Anastomosis between bowel and bile ducts (on CT scan)
E	Endoscopic retrograde cholangiopancreatography (ERCP)	History of recent ERCP
I	Infection (emphysematous cholecystitis)	Air in the gallbladder, sometimes with air in the bile ducts
C	Chronic pancreatitis	Pancreatic calcification
S	Sphincterotomy	

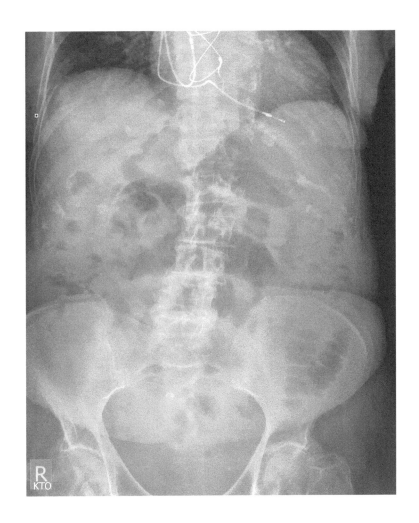

Diagnosis: Gallstone ileus

MODEL ANSWER

This is a plain abdominal radiograph of an adult patient. There is a well-defined branching tubular lucency centred on the right upper quadrant, in keeping with air in the biliary tree. There is moderate dilatation of several loops of small bowel. I cannot see a calcified gallstone within the abdomen. There is no evidence of a pneumoperitoneum.

There are pacemaker leads. The lung bases are unremarkable. There is no bony abnormality.

In summary, there is pneumobilia with small bowel dilatation. This is most likely to represent a gallstone ileus, even without the presence of a calcified stone in the lower abdomen. Adhesional small bowel obstruction with a pre-existing sphincterotomy is also possible, but this would need correlation with the clinical history. If there is clinical doubt, a CT scan of the abdomen and pelvis would provide clarification.

Discussion

Air in the biliary tree (pneumobilia) is caused by three mechanisms:

1. fistula between the biliary system and bowel – this may be iatrogenic (biliary-enteric anastomoses) or pathological (gallstone ileus, between the duodenum and gallbladder)
2. dysfunction of the sphincter of Oddi – this may be pathological (scarring from chronic pancreatitis) or iatrogenic (recent ERCP or previous sphincterotomy)
3. infection – particularly emphysematous cholecystitis; the gas is usually centred on the gallbladder and only seen in the biliary tree in a minority of cases.

You should be able to distinguish pneumobilia from portal venous gas easily on a CT scan. However, they can appear similar on a plain film. Air in the biliary tree classically appears as central branching linear lucencies, which do not reach the liver edge. The central location of the gas is related to the direction of flow of the bile. Portal venous gas is also seen as branching linear lucencies, but these are nearer to the periphery of the liver (classically within 2 cm), which is also to do with the direction of flow of the portal venous blood. A serious cause of portal venous gas is mesenteric infarction. This condition usually has a very poor prognosis. Therefore, it is vital that you try to differentiate between these two pathologies, not just for the exam but also in your clinical practice.

Gallstone ileus is rare but can result in a clear triad of signs on a plain abdominal radiograph or CT scan (Rigler's triad). It therefore appears far more commonly in the exam setting than in real life. The signs are partial or complete bowel obstruction (usually small bowel), gas in the biliary tree and an ectopic calcified gallstone. The calcified gallstone is usually 2.5 cm or larger, commonly lies within the terminal ileum and is therefore seen in the lower abdomen or pelvis on a radiograph. Unfortunately, the majority of gallstones are not calcified and will not be seen on plain radiography. Even without an obvious focus of lower abdominal calcification, gallstone ileus remains the most likely diagnosis when pneumobilia is seen together with small bowel dilatation. The other causes of air in the biliary tree are not usually associated with bowel obstruction (adhesions after biliary-enteric surgery is a possible, but rare, alternative cause).

Pearls

- If you spot some pneumobilia in an exam film, your reflex should be to search for features of gallstone ileus.
- Pneumobilia, small bowel dilatation and a lower abdominal focal calcification (i.e. Rigler's triad) indicate gallstone ileus.
- Pneumobilia can be distinguished from portal venous gas by its central position and the absence of lucencies in the periphery of the liver – remember, the gas "goes with the flow".

31.
Terminal ileal mass/stricture

"TLC"

	Condition	Associated features
T	TB	Non-specific – cannot be reliably differentiated from Crohn's disease Most commonly ileocaecal involvement Narrowed, thick-walled, cone-shaped caecum CT: pericaecal lymphadenopathy – nodes have low attenuation necrotic centres
L	Lymphoma	Non-specific small bowel involvement Nodular, diffuse bowel wall thickening/ulceration Luminal narrowing Aneurysmal dilatation of bowel Polyps – may cause intussusception if large CT: variable – bowel wall thickening, mesenteric masses, lymphadenopathy
C	Crohn's disease	Terminal ileal involvement in the majority of cases Skip lesions Aphthous ulceration (irregular pools of barium) "Rose-thorn" and "cobblestone" ulceration Asymmetrical mucosal involvement – commonly at the mesenteric border, which can lead to pseudosacculations Fistulae (to bladder, bowel, skin) Intra-abdominal abscesses Strictures Separation of bowel loops – bowel wall thickening or fatty hypertrophy

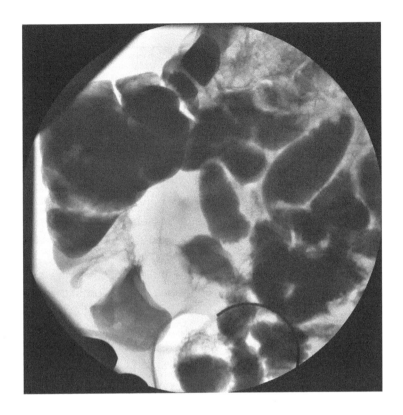

Diagnosis: Crohn's disease

MODEL ANSWER

This is a single spot film from a small bowel follow-through examination. There is circumferential narrowing of the terminal ileum. If this is a permanent feature, that does not dilate normally on subsequent images, it would be in keeping with a terminal ileal stricture.

The medial wall of the caecum, adjacent to the ileocaecal valve, demonstrates an irregular "cobblestone" mucosal pattern. The caecal pole appears normal, as does the remainder of the visible small and large bowel.

In summary, there is a stricture of the terminal ileum and "cobblestone" mucosa within the caecum. These features suggest Crohn's disease. The differential diagnoses include tuberculosis and small bowel lymphoma.

To take this further, I would review the remaining images of this small bowel follow-through series to assess for skip lesions, separation of the small bowel loops or other features that would support the diagnosis of Crohn's disease. I would also review the clinical history and any previous imaging. If Crohn's is suspected and the patient is acutely unwell, a CT scan of the abdomen and pelvis would be useful to identify any abscesses or fistulae.

Discussion

When you are presented with a single image from a barium series, it is important to understand that this is a snapshot of a dynamic study. Apparent strictures seen on one image may not be present on subsequent images, as they were only ever due to peristalsis. This would be obvious if you were performing the test yourself. Therefore, during your presentation, it is recommended that you check whether the changes seen on any single image are permanent. Some candidates may directly ask the examiner if this is the case ("Can I assume this is a constant feature?"). However, we favour including a suitable statement in your description or summary, as in the model answer presented here. This will save you time (as you will not need to wait for the examiner's response) and you will not run the risk of annoying your examiner.

Crohn's disease is a chronic relapsing inflammatory disorder of the gastrointestinal tract that predominantly affects the small bowel and colon. It commonly presents at a young age. It is characterised by erosions, ulceration and full thickness bowel wall inflammation. The involvement of the bowel is often segmental and interspersed with regions of normal bowel. This finding is characteristic and known as skip lesions.

Imaging of the small bowel in inflammatory bowel disease is usually achieved with a small bowel follow-through study, as in this case. MRI of the small bowel is now developing into the modality of choice for the follow-up of young patients with established inflammatory bowel disease. MRI can more readily assess for active disease (bowel wall oedema and classically stratified wall enhancement), strictures and extraluminal disease such as fistulae and abscess formation without the use of ionising radiation. We do not expect that you will be given a small bowel MR image to read in the exam. However, it is worth having a basic knowledge of this test, should the subject arise during discussion of a Crohn's case.

Pearls

- Crohn's disease is a transmural inflammatory disease, characterised by skip lesions, deep fissures, a "cobblestone" mucosal pattern of ulceration, fistulae, sinus tracts, abscesses and strictures.
- On CT, small bowel wall thickening (oedema or mural fat), proliferation of the mesenteric fat (causing separation of small bowel loops) and prominent mesenteric vessels ("comb" sign) is suggestive of Crohn's.
- Post-radiation and ischaemic strictures are also on the differential list of diagnoses and could be mentioned if the examiner asks, "Are there any other causes?"

"INR"

	Condition	Associated features
I	Inflammatory (ulcerative colitis [UC]/Crohn's disease) Infective (pseudomembranous) Ischaemic	UC: • continuous disease extending proximally from rectum, no skip lesions • small bowel normal, except in "backwash" ileitis • symmetrical mucosal involvement • granular mucosa • progressive loss of haustral pattern over time • "lead pipe" colon if chronic • pseudopolyps (islands of normal mucosa) • dilated transverse colon with "thumbprinting" (toxic megacolon) Crohn's disease: • skip lesions • most commonly terminal ileal involvement • aphthous ulceration (irregular pools of barium) • "rose-thorn" and "cobblestone" ulceration • asymmetrical mucosal involvement – commonly mesenteric border, which can lead to pseudosacculations • fistulae (to bladder, bowel, skin) • intra-abdominal abscesses • strictures • separation of bowel loops – bowel wall thickening or fatty hypertrophy Infective (pseudomembranous colitis): • non-specific findings will vary • bowel wall thickening, "thumbprinting" • pericolic fat stranding • bowel dilatation, pneumoperitoneum (on abdominal radiograph [AXR]) • "accordion" sign (on CT) • often left colon, but whole colon may be involved

	Condition	Associated features
I	(cont.)	Ischaemic: ● most commonly around splenic flexure ● may see "thumbprinting" on AXR, segmental bowel wall thickening on CT, if acute ● may see strictures on barium enema, if chronic
N	Neoplastic (especially lymphoma) Neutropenic	Neoplastic: ● non-specific ● wall thickening, luminal narrowing, strictures ● adjacent enlarged lymph nodes Neutropenic (typhlitis): wall thickening and pericolic inflammation of caecum ± ascending colon
R	Radiation	Non-specific Confined to the radiation field, e.g. rectosigmoid with a history of radiotherapy for prostatic/cervical carcinoma

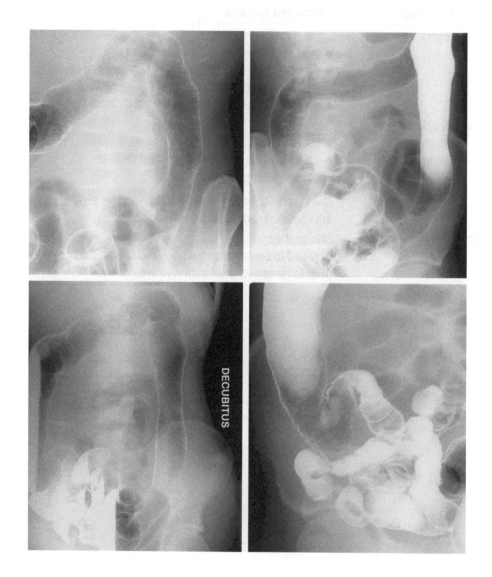

Diagnosis: UC with a proximal transverse colon carcinoma

MODEL ANSWER

These are selected images from a double-contrast barium enema examination. The whole colon, including the rectum, is ahaustral and shortened, with a diffusely granular mucosal pattern. There are no colonic strictures.

There is distortion of the ileocaecal valve, which must be incompetent as the contrast refluxes into the terminal ileum. The terminal ileum adjacent to the ileocaecal valve is dilated and also has a granular mucosal pattern. The more proximal terminal ileum appears normal, with a normal calibre lumen and no strictures demonstrated.

There is a well-defined soft tissue mass within the proximal transverse colon, seen on two of the available images.

The visible bony structures appear normal.

In summary, there is a long-standing pancolitis involving the rectum and extending into the terminal ileum through a distorted and incompetent ileocaecal valve. There is also a mass arising within the transverse colon. The features are of ulcerative colitis with "backwash" ileitis, and a possible colonic carcinoma.

To take this further, I would refer the patient to the colorectal surgeons. If a transverse colon tumour is confirmed at endoscopy, a staging CT scan of the chest, abdomen and pelvis should be performed.

Discussion

Colitis may be seen in the examination on a plain abdominal radiograph, barium enema (as in this case) or abdominal CT scans. Except for clear cases of UC and Crohn's disease, the imaging findings in colitis are often non-specific.

On AXR, "thumbprinting" is a classic sign – the thickening of large bowel haustrations that project into the gas-filled lumen. Any type of colitis can cause this. It would be sensible to mention inflammatory bowel disease, infection and ischaemia as being the most likely causes.

Inflammatory bowel disease is associated with sacroiliitis. Crohn's disease can be associated with gallstones. These are classic secondary signs to look for specifically on both the plain AXR and double-contrast barium enema.

Double-contrast barium enema examinations provide excellent visualisation of the mucosa in inflammatory bowel disease. It is important to be able to spot the different types of mucosal abnormality, as listed here, to help you to distinguish between Crohn's disease and UC. The distribution of disease is also particularly helpful. UC will involve the rectum and a variable amount of contiguous large bowel proximally. Crohn's disease will often involve the terminal ileum and right colon with intervening segments of normal bowel (skip lesions). Ischaemic colitis classically involves the splenic flexure, as this is the watershed area between the superior and inferior mesenteric artery territories. Typhlitis is classically seen in the caecum and ascending colon, occurring in immunocompromised or neutropenic patients undergoing treatment for malignancy.

"Backwash" ileitis is associated with UC. Features to look for include a patulous ileocaecal valve and a dilated terminal ileum with a granular mucosal pattern, as in this case. The length of ileum affected can vary from 5 to 25 cm.

Long-standing UC is associated with an increased risk of developing colonic carcinoma, as in this case – therefore, scrutinise the film for a tumour.

Pearls

- The three "I's" – inflammation, infection and ischaemia – are the top three differential diagnoses for colitis.
- UC is associated with toxic megacolon and increased risk of colonic carcinoma.
- Crohn's disease is associated with skip lesions, terminal ileal involvement, fistulae and intra-abdominal abscesses.
- On AXR, look for "thumbprinting" and associated sacroiliitis, gallstones or pneumoperitoneum.
- On barium enema, also look for evidence of colonic malignancy in cases of long-standing colitis.
- Focal inflammation/stricturing at the splenic flexure of the colon is suggestive of ischaemic colitis.

33.
Solid mesenteric/ peritoneal mass

	Condition	Associated features
L	Lymphoma	Multiple masses Ill-defined confluent mass that encases structures but does not usually compress them Retroperitoneal lymph nodes Splenomegaly
C	Carcinoid	Mass with focal calcifications within a thickened mesentery Stellate radiating pattern within surrounding mesentery (desmoplastic reaction) Tethering of small bowel loops Enhancing small bowel mass (the primary lesion) Hypervascular liver metastases
F	Fibromatosis (desmoid)	Predominantly solid, soft tissue attenuation Well defined Retraction of the associated bowel Associated with Gardner's syndrome: • subcutaneous nodules • multiple colonic polyps • skull and mandibular osteomas • other soft tissue tumours
M	Metastases	Evidence of primary tumour Lymphadenopathy, which may be localised
S	Sclerosing mesenteritis Sarcoma	Sclerosing mesenteritis: • similar in appearance to carcinoid • retraction and calcification Sarcoma: • rare • variable appearances

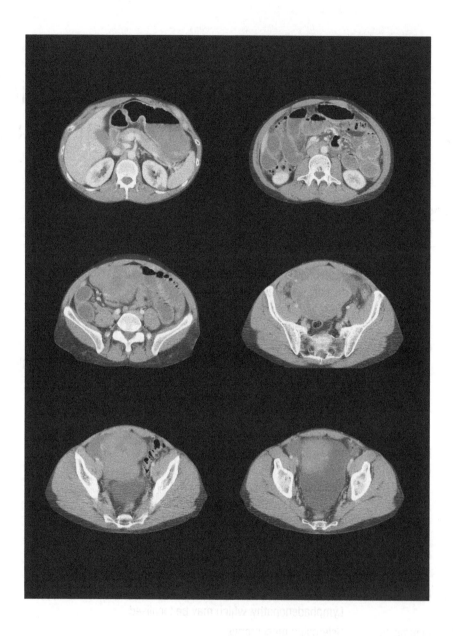

Diagnosis: Desmoid tumour

MODEL ANSWER

These are selected axial CT images of the abdomen and pelvis, with IV contrast in the portal venous phase, of an adult patient. There is a large, solid, well-defined mass in the anterior lower abdomen and pelvis. It does not appear to arise from bowel or the adnexal structures, suggesting a probable mesenteric origin. There is no discernable calcification, fat or cystic component within it. There is no obvious desmoplastic reaction of the mesentery. It abuts the anterior abdominal wall. The mass compresses the distal small bowel, resulting in dilatation of proximal small bowel loops. There is no hydronephrosis. The intra-abdominal viscera otherwise appear unremarkable. No lymphadenopathy is apparent.

In summary, there is a large mesenteric mass in the lower abdomen and pelvis that is compressing the small bowel, causing a degree of obstruction. There is a wide list of possible differential diagnoses, which include lymphoma, carcinoid, desmoid, sarcoma and a large metastasis or a chronic inflammatory mass.

To take this further, I would review the clinical history and other available imaging. I would arrange for the patient to be discussed at the next gastrointestinal MDT meeting. An ultrasound-guided biopsy could be performed to obtain histology.

Discussion

When considering a large abdominal mass, it is important to have a checklist of features to consider when thinking aloud in the viva setting. Answer the following questions in your response:

- Where is it?
- Is it well or ill-defined?
- Is it solid, cystic, fatty or a combination of these?
- Is there any calcification?
- Is there invasion or compression of adjacent structures; for example, hydronephrosis, bowel obstruction or vascular invasion?
- Are there other masses or a primary tumour?

In this case, there is a large mesenteric mass causing small bowel obstruction. There are no particular features to indicate the likely diagnosis, but carcinoid would less likely be due to the absence of calcification and desmoplastic reaction. Therefore, a good knowledge of the possible differential diagnoses is important.

Pearls

- When confronted with a large mesenteric mass, look for calcification within the mass, other masses, liver metastases and retroperitoneal lymph nodes to narrow the list of differential diagnoses.
- Mentioning MDT discussion and consideration of image-guided biopsy indicates knowledge of good practice.

34

Renal papillary necrosis

"ADIOS"

	Condition(s)	Associated feature
A	Analgesics (especially non-steroidal anti-inflammatory drugs) Alcohol	Analgesics: • occasional renal papillary calcification (may be ring-shaped) • signs of painful conditions requiring analgesic use include "bamboo spine", sacroiliitis, sacroiliac joint ankylosis, femoral head osteonecrosis, advanced osteoarthritis
D	Diabetes	Vascular calcification
I	Infection	May be unilateral
O	Obstruction	Renal/ureteric stones May be unilateral
S	Sickle cell disease	Bone infarcts Gallstones Small, calcified or absent spleen Osteonecrosis of femoral heads H-shaped vertebrae

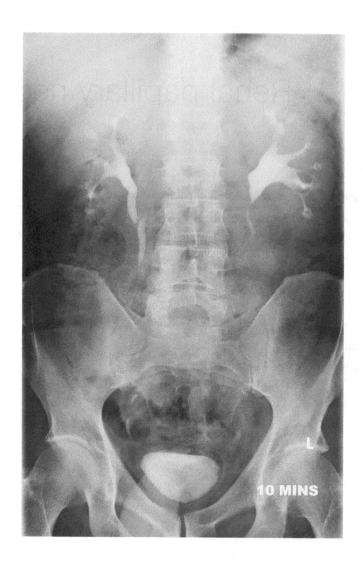

Diagnosis: Analgesic nephropathy

MODEL ANSWER

This is a single image from an IVU [intravenous urography] series, acquired 10 minutes post-contrast administration. It would be my normal practice to review the control film for pathology obscured by the contrast medium.

(You are told that the control is non-contributory.)

Contrast is seen in both pelvicalcyeal systems, ureters and within the bladder, with no evidence of renal tract obstruction. The collecting systems of both kidneys are abnormal, with lateral and central extensions of contrast from the renal fornices into the papillae giving an "egg-in-cup" appearance. No sloughed papillae are visible.

The vertebral column, visualised pelvis and femoral heads appear normal. There are no calcified gallstones and the spleen has a normal outline.

The findings are of bilateral renal papillary necrosis. There are no features on this film to indicate the underlying cause. The differential diagnoses include diabetes, excessive analgesic use, sickle cell disease and infection.

To take this further, I would correlate these findings with the patient's clinical history and review any available previous imaging. If this is a new finding, I would refer the patient to a renal physician for follow-up.

Discussion

Renal papillary necrosis (RPN) is a reasonably common exam case. Most candidates will spot RPN on an IVU image, but to gain full marks in the examination you will need to search for the secondary signs that will provide the diagnosis. When associated with a "bamboo spine" and fused sacroiliac joints, RPN is likely to be due to analgesic nephropathy resulting from painful ankylosing spondylitis. A patient with RPN and H-shaped or biconcave vertebral bodies is likely to have sickle cell disease. The above are likely exam scenarios, but be prepared for other permutations that could occur.

RPN can have a variety of appearances on IVU. All of these involve an abnormal appearance to the renal fornix (the inner border of a calyx where it meets the papilla). The normal calyx – outlined by contrast on the excretory phase of an IVU – has the shape of a shallow cup. Defects in the fornix can extend into the papilla either centrally ("egg-in-cup", as in this case), peripherally ("lobster claw"), or peripherally and circumferentially to detach the papilla ("signet ring"). A detached papilla may remain in situ and calcify or move, leaving a round, blunted, ball-shaped calyx. If calyces are blunted, look for sloughed papillae within the collecting systems and ureters, as these can cause ureteric obstruction.

Pearls

- *Always* ask for the control film when presented with a post-contrast IVU image – there may be underlying calculi obscured by contrast.
- Be aware of the various appearances of RPN on IVU: abnormal streaks of contrast from the fornices, "lobster claw", ring shadows, "egg-in-cup", deformed calyces and sloughed papillae.
- Once confident of RPN, look at the underlying bones of lumbar vertebrae, pelvis and femoral heads. Is there any sign of sickle cell disease, ankylosing spondylitis, severe femoral head osteoarthosis or orthopaedic surgery?
- There may be no features to indicate an underlying diagnosis, so suggest correlation with the clinical history for analgesic use, diabetes and previous urology admissions for pyelonephritis or renal colic.

35.
Nephrocalcinosis

"Medics Hate Renal Calculi"

	Condition	Associated features
M	Medullary sponge kidney	Normal biochemistry "Paintbrush" or "bunch-of-flowers" appearance on IVU Kidney may be enlarged
H	Hyperparathyroidism (primary) Hyperoxaluria (rare)	Hyperparathyroidism: • serum calcium and phosphate abnormalities • bone resorption • osteosclerosis • brown tumours • soft tissue calcification Hyperoxaluria: • dense homogenous nephrogram on plain film • osteopenia and other skeletal abnormalities • may present in childhood and have a renal transplant
R	Renal tubular acidosis	Metabolic acidosis Osteopenia, fractures, Looser's zones Most common cause of nephrocalcinosis in childhood
C	Calcium excess (sarcoid, vitamin D excess, immobilisation)	Rare causes of nephrocalcinosis

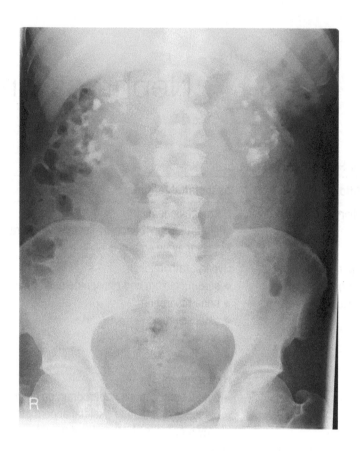

Diagnosis: Renal tubular acidosis

Definition: Diffuse calcification within the renal parenchyma, distinct from the renal calculi, seen within the pelvicalyceal systems and ureters

---

MODEL ANSWER

This is a plain abdominal radiograph of an adult patient. There are large clusters of discrete calcification within the renal pyramids bilaterally. There are no ureteric calculi. The bones are of normal density with no areas of lysis or sclerosis.

In summary, there is bilateral medullary nephrocalcinosis. The most common causes of this are hyperparathyroidism, medullary sponge kidney and renal tubular acidosis.

To take this further, I would review any relevant previous imaging. If available, I would review hand radiographs to look for evidence of phalangeal resorption suggestive of hyperparathyroidism. I would also review any previous IVU series to look for evidence of contrast pooling in the papillae, which would be suggestive of medullary sponge kidney.

A review of the clinical history and recent biochemistry results, especially calcium, phosphate and pH levels, would also be useful. Medullary sponge kidney would be likely if the patient were asymptomatic with no biochemical abnormality.

Discussion

An exam case of medullary nephrocalcinosis could also manifest as a selection of abdominal ultrasound images that would show diffusely echogenic renal pyramids. An IVU or CT study is also possible. The main aim is to concisely identify and describe the abnormality and name the three most likely diagnoses, as in the model answer provided. It would be difficult to establish the exact diagnosis based on plain radiography alone; biochemistry and patient history would be helpful in discriminating between the diagnoses.

Both nephrocalcinosis and renal stones can be seen in a proportion of patients with primary hyperparathyroidism (rarely in secondary). A film showing nephrocalcinosis in this patient group may show the other recognised skeletal features of hyperparathyroidism (see table).

Medullary sponge kidney is a congenital cystic dilatation of the collecting ducts, which frequently contain small calculi. It may affect only one kidney or even only a focal area of a single kidney. On IVU, there is often the classic finding of "paintbrush" striations resulting from pooling of contrast within these cystic dilatations. Patients with medullary sponge kidney are often asymptomatic, but there is an association with renal calculi and recurrent urinary tract infection. Blood tests are usually normal.

Renal tubular acidosis (type 1) is a failure of the kidney to excrete acid, resulting in metabolic acidosis. The associated hypercalcinuria causes nephrocalcinosis and renal calculi. This condition is associated with osteomalacia. Therefore, possible secondary features to look out for on a film demonstrating evidence of nephrocalcinosis include osteopenia, vertebral fractures and Looser's zones.

Hyperoxaluria is a rare autosomal recessive enzyme deficiency resulting in oxalate deposition in the kidneys and may present in childhood. Plain abdominal radiographs may show diffusely dense bilateral renal outlines – like a nephrogram but without the contrast. It is associated with skeletal abnormalities, particularly osteopenia. There is progressive renal dysfunction that may necessitate renal transplantation.

Pearls

- Be able to recite the top three causes of nephrocalcinosis: hyperparathyroidism, medullary sponge kidney and renal tubular acidosis.
- Look for bony abnormalities such as osteopenia, osteosclerosis, brown tumours and Looser's zones.
- While biochemistry results are a helpful discriminator, remember this is a radiology exam, so discuss the radiology first. Medullary sponge kidney is not associated with abnormality of electrolyte, pH, calcium or phosphate serum levels and can be an incidental finding.
- Be aware of the rarer causes of nephrocalcinosis.

Section 4

Neuroradiology

36

Single or multiple ring-enhancing brain lesions

"MAGIC DR"

	Condition	Associated features
M	Metastasis	Multiple or solitary Significant surrounding oedema Commonly at grey–white matter junction Most common infratentorial mass in an adult Thick and irregular wall (compared with an abscess)
A	Abscess	Usually solitary Smooth thin walls with uniform enhancement Restricted diffusion on MRI Significant surrounding oedema
G	Glioma	Usually solitary but sometimes multifocal May be large with irregular outline Irregular nodular ring enhancement Significant surrounding oedema (if high-grade) Mass effect Crossing the midline via corpus callosum is suggestive Commonly in the deep white matter
I	Infarct	Corresponds to vascular territories Modest enhancement if subacute
C	Contusion	A rare cause Associated haemorrhage, skull fracture, coup and contrecoup injuries
D	Demyelination	Acute demyelinating plaques may demonstrate incomplete ring enhancement
R	Radiation	Possible evidence of previous surgery

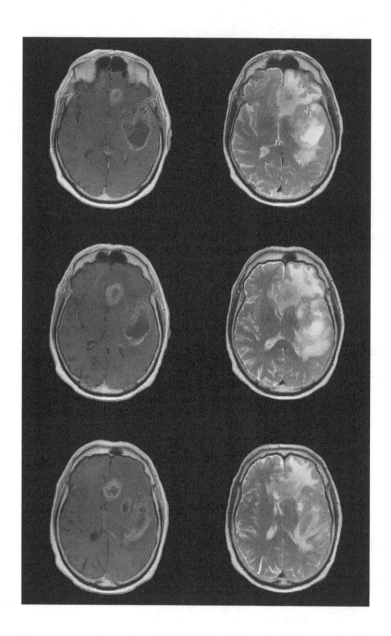

Diagnosis: Multifocal glioblastoma multiforme (GBM)

MODEL ANSWER

These are selected axial T2 and T1 post-contrast images of the brain of an adult patient. There are three intra-axial mass lesions. Two are within the white matter of left temporoparietal lobes. The third lesion is within the left medial frontal lobe and extends across the midline via the genu of the corpus callosum. These lesions are mixed solid and cystic and demonstrate avid irregular ring enhancement. There is a large amount of adjacent vasogenic oedema. The lesions show mass effect, with effacement of the lateral ventricles and midline shift to the right. There is no hydrocephalus.

In summary, there are three supratentorial ring-enhancing lesions. The most likely cause is a multifocal glioma, metastases or abscess. The large size and irregularity of the left temporal lesion as well as the smaller lesion crossing the midline favour multifocal glioma.

To take this further, I would review the diffusion-weighted images. Restricted diffusion would favour the diagnosis of abscesses. A CT scan of the chest, abdomen and pelvis could be arranged to look for a primary malignancy or source of infection. I would urgently refer the patient to the local neurosurgical unit for further assessment.

Discussion

The "MAGIC DR" mnemonic can apply to single or multiple ring-enhancing lesions. Ring-enhancing brain lesions are commonly seen in daily practice and therefore also in the exam. It is a particularly good mnemonic, as the first three letters refer to the three most common causes of a ring-enhancing brain lesion.

It may be difficult to distinguish between metastasis, abscess and glioma on contrast-enhanced CT images and MRI. However, the presence of restricted diffusion – high signal diffusion-weighted imaging (DWI) with corresponding low signal apparent diffusion coefficient (ADC) – strongly suggests a bacterial abscess. It would therefore be useful to ask to see diffusion-weighted images if not immediately available. In terms of differentiating primary and secondary brain malignancy, several factors are useful. A large mass with irregular enhancement suggests a glioma. A lesion that crosses the midline is also suggestive of a primary tumour, classically GBM or lymphoma. Multifocal glioma can occur in a minority of patients, as in this case, but there will rarely be more than three separate lesions. When multiple, small well-defined ring-enhancing lesions are seen at the grey–white matter junction, these are likely to represent metastases. The presence of significant oedema and mass effect can be seen in all three of these pathologies, and does not aid in differentiating between them.

Pearls

- Metastasis, abscess and glioma are the most likely causes.
- Multiple ring-enhancing lesions suggest metastases.
- A large, irregularly shaped lesion that demonstrates ring enhancement and crosses the midline is suggestive of a glioma.
- Lung, breast and melanoma are the primary tumours most commonly associated with brain metastases.
- Restricted diffusion strongly suggests a bacterial abscess.
- Good management steps include clinical correlation; obtaining a CT scan of the chest, abdomen and pelvis to identify a primary tumour or source of sepsis; and urgently seeking neurosurgical opinion.
- Consider toxoplasmosis in the HIV-positive patient with ring-enhancing lesions centred on the basal ganglia.

37.
Cerebellopontine angle mass

"SAME" or "Not all cerebellopontine angle masses are the SAME"

	Condition	Features
S	Schwannoma (vestibular)	Avid enhancement Intracanalicular component may expand the internal auditory meatus (IAM) Acute angle with petrous temporal bone May be heterogenous if large or have a cystic component
A	Arachnoid cyst	No enhancement Isointense to cerebrospinal fluid (CSF) in all sequences No restricted diffusion
M	Meningioma	Avid enhancement Dural tail Obtuse angle with petrous temporal bone Adjacent hyperostosis Calcifications
E	Epidermoid cyst	No enhancement Isointense to CSF in most sequences Higher signal than CSF on fluid-attenuated inversion recovery (FLAIR) Restricted diffusion

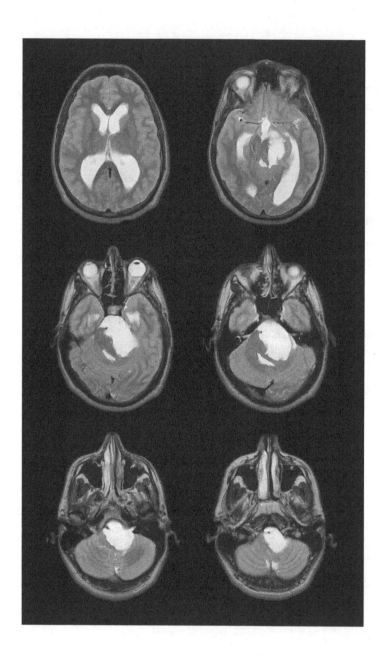

Diagnosis: Epidermoid cyst

MODEL ANSWER

These are selected axial T2-weighted MR images of an adult brain. There is a well-defined mass centred on the left CP [cerebellopontine] angle. This demonstrates homogeneous increased T2 signal, which is isointense to that of the CSF. There is no expansion of the left internal auditory meatus. The mass compresses and displaces the pons to the right. There is mild ventricular dilatation. No intercerebral oedema can be seen.

In summary, there is a large mass centred on the left CP angle of homogeneous CSF intensity. This most likely represents a long-standing epidermoid cyst or an arachnoid cyst. The homogenous fluid signal makes the diagnosis of schwannoma or meningioma less likely.

It would be my normal practice to obtain and review post-contrast and diffusion-weighted images for evidence of enhancement and restricted diffusion.

(Further DWI and post-contrast images are then shown.)

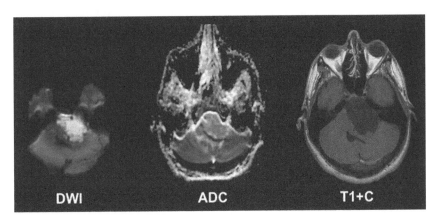

These are selected DWI, ADC and post-contrast axial images at the level of the cerebellopontine angle. The mass demonstrates restricted diffusion but does not enhance. The features are of an epidermoid cyst.

Discussion

Most (80%–90%) CP angle masses are schwannomas, while most of the rest are meningiomas. Epidermoid cysts (the third most common CP angle mass) and bilateral vestibular schwannomas appear more commonly in the exam setting than in clinical practice, reflecting their potential to test your observational skills and knowledge.

Both schwannomas and meningiomas enhance avidly. Schwannomas frequently widen the IAM whereas meningiomas do not. The presence of a heterogenous signal (from cysts or haemorrhage) suggests schwannoma. Calcification and a broad dural base suggest meningioma. The angle that the mass forms with the petrous temporal bone is also a discriminator between these two lesions.

Epidermoid cysts are more common than arachnoid cysts in this location. Neither enhance and only epidermoid cysts demonstrate restricted diffusion (high DWI signal with corresponding low ADC signal). Therefore, it is important to see post-contrast and diffusion-weighted sequences when assessing these lesions for the first time.

Bilateral eighth cranial nerve (acoustic) schwannomas are pathognomonic for neurofibromatosis type 2 (NF-2). This is a classic exam case. Always mention the association with other schwannomas (such as those of the facial nerve), meningiomas and ependymomas and look for multiple tumours of the brain and spinal cord. The majority of NF-2 patients also have spinal cord tumours. Therefore, if you make this diagnosis in the exam from an MR image of the brain only, you should suggest that an MRI of the whole spine should be performed as part of your further management.

Pearls

- Establish that the mass is centred on the CP angle.
- Note the shape, signal characteristics, homogeneity, extension into IAM and effect upon local structures.
- Ask for post-gadolinium and diffusion-weighted images if they are not provided.
- Enhancement favours schwannoma or meningioma. Use the criteria given in the table to establish which is most likely.
- Bilateral CP angle acoustic schwannomas are pathognomonic for NF-2. Look for other brain tumours and ask to review contrast-enhanced MRI of the whole spine.
- Epidermoid and arachnoid cysts do not enhance.
- Restricted diffusion is characteristic of an epidermoid cyst.

38

Pituitary region mass

"CAR MAG"

	Condition	Associated features
C	Craniopharyngioma	Most commonly a suprasellar mass Intrasellar extension may occur Peak incidence in childhood and the fifth decade Multilobulated heterogeneous mass containing solid and cystic elements with calcification Variable T1 and T2 signal Vivid enhancement of solid components
A	Adenoma of the pituitary (micro- and macro-)	Microadenoma: ● <10 mm in diameter ● displaces the pituitary gland ● enhances later than the normal pituitary gland Macroadenoma: ● >10 mm in diameter ● centred on intrasellar region, extending into the suprasellar cistern ● expansion of the pituitary fossa ● may invade the cavernous sinus and encase the internal carotid artery ● homogeneous enhancement ● calcification rare ● may haemorrhage or contain cysts
R	Rathke's cleft cyst	Intrasellar, with or without suprasellar extension – a purely suprasellar mass is very rare Thin-walled cyst No calcifications No enhancement, but surrounding normal pituitary tissue may mimic wall enhancement Variable MR signal – may show high (proteinaceous fluid) or low T1 signal

	Condition	Associated features
M	Meningioma Metastasis	Meningioma: • more commonly parasellar/suprasellar than intrasellar • usually solid (may contain cysts) • dural tail • uniform enhancement Metastasis: • rare • often from breast or lung carcinoma • evidence of other metastatic disease/known primary tumour • enhancement • may be indistinguishable from macroadenoma
A	Aneurysm	Flow void on MRI
G	Glioma	Suprasellar Optic chiasm and nerve gliomas are associated with NF-1 Usually enhance

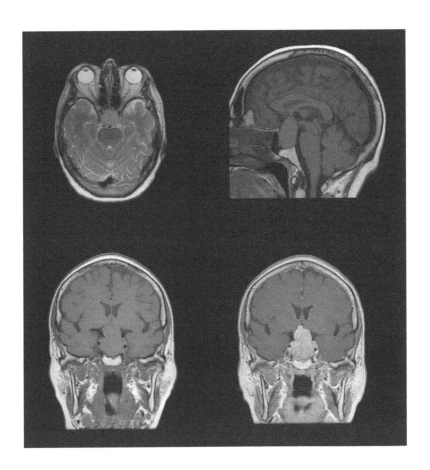

Diagnosis: Pituitary macroadenoma

Definition: A mass situated within one or more of the sellar, parasellar and suprasellar regions

---

MODEL ANSWER

These are selected MR images of an adult brain. The sequences shown are an axial T2, a sagittal T1 and pre- and post-contrast coronal T1 images.

There is a large mass in the pituitary region. The mass arises from and expands the sella, and extends into the suprasellar cistern. The lesion is of homogeneous soft tissue signal. When compared with the normal spinal cord, it is mildly T2 hyperintense and T1 isointense. There are no cysts or calcifications. There is uniform avid enhancement of the mass. On the post-contrast images, the mass extends into both cavernous sinuses and encases the left internal carotid artery.

In summary, there is a homogeneous enhancing intrasellar mass with suprasellar and intracavernous extension. The appearances are in keeping with a pituitary macroadenoma.

To take this further, I would review previous imaging and arrange for the patient to be discussed in the next neurosurgical MDT meeting.

Discussion

A good knowledge of the anatomy of the pituitary region will allow you to describe the epicentre of a pituitary region mass. This will help you to narrow the list of differential diagnoses. The signal and heterogeneity of the mass, enhancement pattern and effect on adjacent structures should also be described. This case is a very typical macroadenoma, centred on the sella with suprasellar and parasellar extension. A Rathke's cleft cyst is also most likely to be centred within the sella but does not enhance. A craniopharyngioma is most likely to be centred in the suprasellar region. Lesions centred lateral to the sella could be any of the other lesions listed in the table.

Pituitary macroadenomas are larger than 10 mm in diameter, while pituitary microadenomas are smaller than 10 mm. The presenting symptoms of these lesions can be partially related to their size. Macroadenomas are hormonally inactive but commonly present as a result of mass effect. For example, suprasellar extension may cause compression of the optic chiasm resulting in bitemporal hemianopia. Microadenomas are hormonally active and often associated with elevated prolactin levels.

When assessing post-contrast images of a suspected pituitary microadenoma, remember that it enhances later than the normal pituitary gland. It will therefore be low signal on the post-contrast T1 images, which seems counterintuitive when thinking about intracranial masses.

Pearls

- First, identify the pituitary gland and sella and note the epicentre of the lesion in relation to these.
- Determine whether the sella is normal or expanded.
- Coronal, axial and sagittal sequences are necessary to assess whether there is involvement of adjacent structures.
- Look for involvement of the cavernous sinus, optic chiasm, optic nerves, hypothalamus and third ventricle.
- An expansile mass centred within the sella is most likely to be a pituitary macroadenoma.
- A mass with a suprasellar epicentre, cysts and calcifications is most likely to be a craniopharyngioma.
- A cystic pituitary region mass, with no or minimal rim enhancement, is most likely to be a Rathke's cleft cyst.

39.
Basal ganglia calcification

"Normal BIRTH"

	Condition	Associated features
Normal	Normal variant	Usually in the globus pallidus bilaterally Not usually extensive
B	Birth anoxia/hypoxia	Variable calcification
I	Infection – congenital (toxoplasmosis) Inherited (Fahr's disease)	Toxoplasmosis: ● scattered focal irregular and/or curvilinear calcifications involving basal ganglia ● hydrocephalus ● abnormal brain parenchyma Inherited: bilateral extensive calcification
R	Radiotherapy	Evidence of previous surgery Encephalomalacia
T	Toxins (carbon monoxide, lead)	
H	Hypocalcaemia	Bilateral extensive calcification

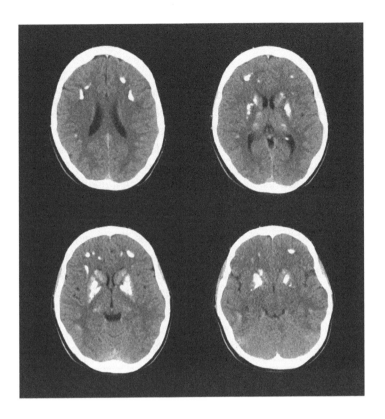

Diagnosis: Congenital hypocalcaemia (pseudohypoparathyroidism)

MODEL ANSWER

These are selected axial images from an unenhanced CT scan of the brain in an adult patient. There is extensive focal calcification within the brain parenchyma. This has a symmetrical distribution, which is primarily centred on the lentiform nuclei but also involves both thalami and caudate heads to a lesser extent. There is further focal calcification within the deep white matter of both frontal lobes. There is no subependymal calcification. No significant cerebral atrophy, oedema or hydrocephalus is evident.

In summary, there is extensive intracerebral calcification primarily involving the basal ganglia and white matter of the frontal lobes. The brain parenchyma otherwise appears normal. This is most likely to represent an inherited disorder such as hypoparathyroidism, pseudohypoparathyroidism or Fahr's disease. If there is a history of malignancy, previous brain radiotherapy could also be a possible cause.

I would correlate these findings with the clinical history and review previous imaging. I would also review recent serum calcium and PTH levels to look for evidence for hypocalcaemia and hypoparathyroidism.

Discussion

Basal ganglia calcification is relatively common, usually idiopathic and an incidental finding on CT scans. The calcification in these cases is not usually extensive, and therefore unlikely to appear in a viva setting. When there is dramatic calcification, as in this case, a reasonable set of diagnoses include metabolic, post-infectious and inherited conditions, as described in the table.

It demonstrates good clinical radiology knowledge to mention that you would like to review serum calcium and PTH levels to look for evidence of hypoparathyroidism. This condition is also typically associated with short fourth and fifth metacarpals, so asking to see a previous hand radiograph would also demonstrate your wider knowledge.

Pearls

- Establish if the calcification is diffuse or where it is centred.
- If the underlying calcification is extensive and relatively symmetrical – consider inherited causes – hypocalcaemia and Fahr's disease. Serum calcium levels would help distinguish the two.
- If the underlying brain is abnormal, displaying hydrocephalus and cortical atrophy, for example, consider congenital TORCH (i.e. toxoplasmosis, other infections, rubella, *Cytomegalovirus*, *Herpes simplex virus 2*) infections.
- Look for signs of malignancy, which may have been treated with radiotherapy.

40.
Intra-axial haemorrhage

"AH, MTV!"

	Condition	Associated features
A	cerebral Amyloid angiopathy	Older age groups Cortical or subcortical location Spares deep white matter, basal ganglia, brainstem Often large haemorrhages Micro-haemorrhages: focal areas of low signal on gradient echo MR sequences Focal areas of encephalomalacia (from previous haemorrhage) Cerebral atrophy and leukoencephalopathy
H	Hypertensive	Commonly in basal ganglia/thalamic location
M	Malignancy	Metastases are more common than primary tumours Metastases are often multiple lesions, at the grey–white matter junction Vasogenic oedema and mass effect Enhancing lesions Primary tumours are usually a single lesion
T	Trauma (contusions)	Small, often multiple parenchymal haemorrhages Especially in inferior frontal lobes and temporal poles – adjacent to bone Signs of trauma: • scalp haematoma • skull fracture • associated extradural/subdural/subarachnoid haemorrhage

	Condition	Associated features
V	Vascular malformation Venous infarction	**Vascular malformation:** ● AVMs – feeding arteries and draining veins post-contrast, nidus of abnormal vessels with calcified foci ● cavernous haemangiomas – "popcorn" appearance on MR with low signal rim, often difficult to see on CT scan **Venous infarction:** ● bilateral parasagittal or bithalamic infarction ± haemorrhage ● temporal lobe infarction ± haemorrhage ● sinus thrombosis – high attenuation in the superior sagittal or transverse sinuses on unenhanced CT, "empty delta" sign on CT venogram

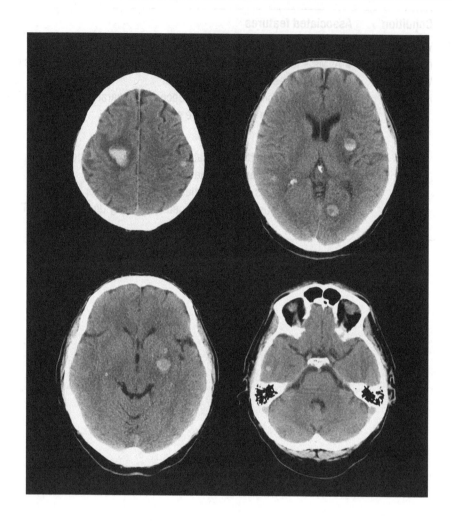

Diagnosis: Melanoma metastases

MODEL ANSWER

These are selected unenhanced CT images of the brain of an adult. There are multiple, well-defined high attenuation lesions predominantly located at the grey–white matter junction. The largest lies in the right centrum semiovale and contains a fluid level. The lesions are surrounded by a moderate amount of vasogenic oedema. There is no significant generalised mass effect or midline shift and no hydrocephalus. There is no obvious evidence of trauma.

In summary, there are multiple haemorrhagic brain lesions. These are most likely to represent metastases. Multiple contusions or bleeding vascular malformations are unlikely. The most common primary tumours to metastasise to the brain are lung and breast carcinoma; however, haemorrhage is also associated with melanoma, renal and thyroid primaries.

To take this further, I would review any previous imaging for evidence of a primary malignancy. In the absence of previous imaging, a CT scan of the chest, abdomen and pelvis as well as triple assessment of the breasts could be performed to identify a primary tumour. Contrast-enhanced MRI would be useful for further characterisation of these lesions.

Discussion

There are several key factors to consider when assessing an intra-axial haemorrhage, which will help to narrow the list of differential diagnoses:

- the number of lesions – multiplicity suggests metastases
- the location – cortical, subcortical (suggests cerebral amyloid angiopathy), grey–white matter junction (suggests metastases), white matter, basal ganglia (suggests hypertensive bleed) or brainstem
- whether there is oedema and mass effect – a disproportionately large amount of oedema when compared with the size of the lesion/s suggests metastases
- whether there is calcification or abnormal vessels within the lesion – suggestive of a vascular malformation
- whether there is haemorrhage within an area of low attenuation – this suggests haemorrhage within an infarct, especially venous infarcts
- whether there is evidence of trauma – this suggests contusions and haematomas.

In this case, multiple well-defined haemorrhagic lesions at the grey–white matter junction are strongly suggestive of metastatic disease. Brain metastases are the most common intracranial tumour in adults. They are usually found at the grey–white matter junction due to the small calibre of vessels in this area. Further evaluation of the brain with contrast-enhanced MRI should be recommended in this situation.

Pearls

- Multiple enhancing lesions, located at the grey–white matter junction, with a disproportionately large amount of surrounding oedema, are suggestive of metastatic disease.
- Lung, breast, melanoma and renal primaries are the most common causes of brain metastases.
- Melanoma, renal cell carcinoma, choriocarcinoma and thyroid carcinoma metastases are associated with haemorrhage (mnemonic = MR CT).
- Melanoma metastases are associated with high T1 signal on MRI due to the presence of melanin.
- Subacute haemorrhage (days to weeks), fat, protein, melanin and gadolinium are well-recognised causes of high T1 signal on MRI.

41

Restricted diffusion in the brain

"SEAL"

	Condition	Associated feature
S	Stroke (acute infarct)	Conforms to an arterial territory Relevant clinical history, acute onset
E	Epidermoid cyst	T2 signal similar to CSF Increased signal on FLAIR No enhancement Most common at the cerebellopontine angles
A	Abscess	Intraparenchymal Peripheral rim enhancement Surrounding vasogenic oedema Mass effect Very low ADC values Relevant clinical history: sepsis and rapid deterioration
L	Lymphoma	Intermediate or low T2 signal relative to grey matter Avid homogenous enhancement May cross midline Relatively little mass effect

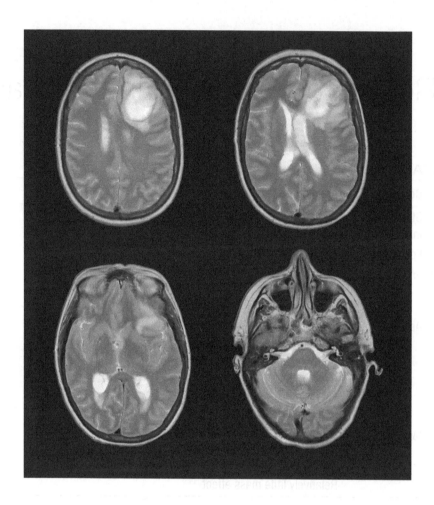

Diagnosis: Cerebral abscess with intraventricular extension

MODEL ANSWER

These are selected axial T2-weighted images of an adult brain. There is a well-defined intra-axial mass within the left frontal lobe, which demonstrates high T2 signal. There is a less well-defined area of increased T2 signal within the white matter surrounding this lesion, in keeping with oedema. The lesion has mass effect causing midline shift to the right. The lesion extends into the left lateral ventricle and there is dependent high signal material within both occipital horns.

In summary, there is an aggressive intra-axial mass within the left frontal lobe with intraventricular extension. If the patient were acutely unwell, I would consider cerebral abscess. If there was a longer history of symptoms, I would also consider a primary brain malignancy or a large cystic metastasis. To take this further, I would like to see contrast-enhanced T1 and diffusion-weighted images to aid further characterisation.

(Images are shown.)

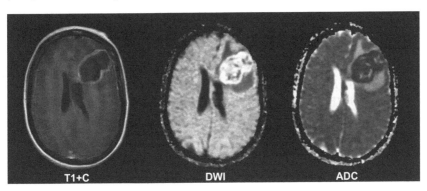

These are selected axial T1 post-contrast, DWI and ADC images of the same patient. The lesion demonstrates peripheral rim enhancement. There is increased DWI signal with corresponding low ADC signal, in keeping with restricted diffusion.

The appearances are of a cerebral abscess. I would inform the local neurosurgical centre and arrange for urgent transfer.

Discussion

Diffusion-weighted MRI assesses the diffusion of water molecules. In practice, three sets of images are obtained: a B0 image, a B1000 image and an ADC map. The B0 image is T2-weighted, with high signal in the ventricles (i.e. CSF), whereas the normal B1000 image has low signal in the CSF spaces. Only the B1000 and ADC images should be scrutinised. Restricted diffusion is characterised by high signal on B1000 (DWI) and corresponding low ADC signal.

DWI is especially useful to differentiate a cerebral abscess from a glioma, and an epidermoid cyst from an arachnoid cyst. GBM and arachnoid cysts do not demonstrate restricted diffusion.

The DWI and ADC signal characteristics of both primary brain tumours and metastases can be variable. However, the presence of restricted diffusion is suggestive of lymphoma, but not a glioma or metastasis.

DWI can provide information about the chronicity of a stroke. Acute infarctions show restricted diffusion but subacute and chronic infarctions do not. The DWI signal will remain high for many months, but the ADC signal will slowly increase with time and become bright at 7–10 days.

Pearls

- Key features to mention with all brain masses are their location, T2 signal intensity, enhancement pattern and associated oedema.
- When shown an MR image of an intracranial mass, consider asking for post-contrast and DWI if they would help to narrow your differential diagnoses.
- For restricted diffusion, look for high DWI signal with corresponding low ADC signal in the region of interest.
- If a lesion is rounded and cystic with surrounding vasogenic oedema, use DWI/ADC to differentiate between an abscess and a necrotic glioma.
- High signal on both DWI and ADC represents "T2 shine through", not restricted diffusion.

42.
Intramedullary spinal mass

"I HEAL"

	Condition	Associated features
I	Infarction	High T2 signal Enhancement not a feature Mild cord expansion in the acute phase, but less so than tumours Restricted diffusion
H	Haemangioblastoma	Usually discrete, avidly enhancing nodules High T2 signal mass Multiple flow voids from vessels Cystic component
E	Ependymoma	Most common spinal tumour in adults Most common in the lumbar spine, conus/filum terminale and cervical spine Well defined Central location in the cord May be heterogeneous with focal cystic change and haemorrhage Well-defined, avid, homogeneous enhancement Bony remodelling is common
A	Astrocytoma	Most common spinal tumour in children but also seen in adults Most commonly found in the thoracic and cervical spine Poorly defined Eccentric location in the cord Bony remodelling not a feature Haemorrhage uncommon

	Condition	Associated features
L	Lipoma (or dermoid cyst)	Both are commonly found in the conus Presentation at >20 years of age Lipoma: • high T1 signal – fat • homogeneous Dermoid: • contains variable proportions of fat, cystic areas and soft tissue components • heterogeneous

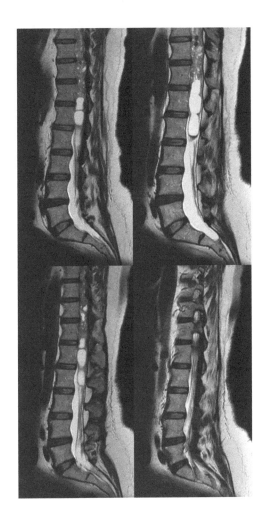

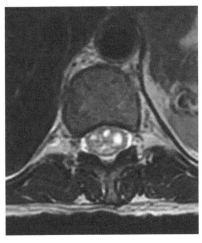

Diagnosis: Ependymoma

MODEL ANSWER

These are selected sagittal T2-weighted images through the lower thoracic and lumbar spine and a single axial T2-weighted image through the lower thoracic spine in an adult patient.

There is an extensive abnormality within the distal spinal cord and conus that extends over a length of at least five vertebral body heights. The lesion expands the spinal cord, in keeping with an intramedullary mass. The lesion also appears centrally placed within the cord, rather than eccentric. It contains focal areas of high and low T2 signal, which may represent cystic change and haemorrhage, but correlation with T1 images is needed. There is a large cystic component at the L1/2 levels.

The bone marrow signal is normal. There is no focal disc lesion. There is no obvious bony remodelling.

In summary, there is an extensive intramedullary spinal cord mass at the thoracolumbar junction involving the conus. In an adult patient, this is most likely to represent an ependymoma. The differential diagnoses include astrocytoma.

To take this further, I would review any relevant previous imaging. If this were a new diagnosis, I would perform a contrast-enhanced MRI of the brain and whole spine to assess for the features of an underlying phakomatosis. I would refer the patient to the neurosurgical team.

Discussion

Intramedullary spinal lesions lie within the substance of the spinal cord. Cord expansion is the key feature of an intramedullary tumour. T2-weighted sequences provide contrast between the cord and the CSF, demonstrating cord expansion nicely.

The most common intramedullary tumour is an ependymoma, followed by astrocytoma. Although there are a few characteristics that may be used to distinguish between these two tumours, it is often impossible to tell them apart using imaging alone. Usefully, the age of the patient may point you towards the most likely diagnosis. Ependymomas are more common in adults, whereas astrocytomas are the most common spinal tumour in children.

Bony remodelling is a useful sign that can be used to help distinguish between an ependymoma and an astrocytoma. Ependymomas are slow-growing tumours with an insidious onset of symptoms including back pain, sensory loss, and bowel and bladder dysfunction. This slow rate of growth is associated with bony remodelling, such as pedicle erosion, laminar thinning and posterior vertebral body scalloping, all of which result in widening of the spinal canal. Conversely, astrocytomas are faster growing tumours and do not typically cause bony remodelling. Scoliosis may be a feature of both tumours.

There is an increased incidence of astrocytomas in NF-1, ependymomas in NF-2 and haemangioblastomas in Von Hippel–Lindau syndrome. These conditions have classical multisystem imaging features, so are seen more often in the exam than in real life. A detailed knowledge of these conditions is essential.

Intramedullary metastases are rare, and therefore not mentioned in this mnemonic. They are more likely to occur when there is disseminated malignancy. They are associated with a disproportionately large area of cord oedema with respect to the size of the lesion.

Pearls

- Mention cord expansion when describing intramedullary spinal tumours.
- Most intramedullary masses are either ependymomas (more common in adults than children) or astrocytomas (more common in children than in adults).
- If the lesion is well defined with areas of cystic change and haemorrhage and there is associated bony remodelling, consider ependymoma.
- Consider astrocytoma if the lesion is ill-defined and eccentrically located.
- Consider possible association with NF-1, NF-2 and Von Hippel–Lindau syndrome.
- Mention that you would perform contrast-enhanced MRI of the brain and whole spine to look for further lesions and the features of phakomatoses such as NF-1.

43.
Extramedullary intradural spinal mass

"No More Spinal Masses"

	Condition	Associated features
N	Neurofibroma	Most commonly found in the cervical spine May be multiple "Dumbbell" appearance if they enter the neural foramen Low T1 and high T2 signal Contrast enhancement "Target" sign on T2-weighted imaging – low signal centre with peripheral high signal (also seen in schwannomas) Haemorrhage and cystic changes are rare Adjacent bony remodelling
M	Meningioma	Usually in thoracic cord (75%) Lateral aspect of cord (90%) Broad-based dural attachment Dural tail Isointense to the cord on T1 and T2 Early avid enhancement
S	Schwannoma	Most commonly found in the cervical and lumbar spine Usually solitary Rounded lesions ± "dumbbell" appearance if they enter the neural foramen Adjacent bony remodelling Low T1 and high T2 signal, contrast enhancement Haemorrhage and cystic changes may occur
M	Metastasis	Commonly multiple, round and of varied sizes Enhancing nodular lesion on the cord and meninges "Sugar coating" of the cord "Drop" metastases – more common in paediatric patients Non-CNS primary tumour – more common in adult patients

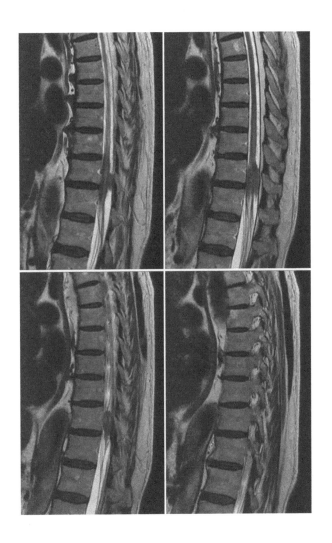

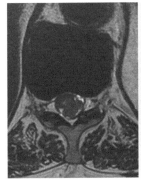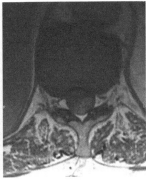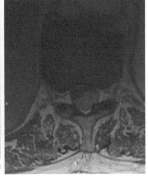

Diagnosis: Melanoma metastasis

MODEL ANSWER

These are selected T2-weighted sagittal images through the thoracolumbar spine with axial T2 and T1 pre- and post-contrast images through a single vertebral level of an adult patient.

There is a focal mass lesion within the spinal canal at the level of the conus medullaris. The lesion is separate from the cord, which it displaces anterolaterally to the right. The lesion is surrounded by CSF, placing it within the dura.

When compared to the spinal cord, the lesion demonstrates moderately high T1 signal, and on T2 sequences is isointense. It enhances homogenously. There is no evidence of adjacent bony remodelling or widening of the neural foramina.

No further mass lesions are demonstrated on the available images.

The bone marrow signal and intervertebral discs are unremarkable.

In summary, there is an intradural extramedullary mass lesion at the level of the conus, which demonstrates increased T1 signal and contrast enhancement. As this is an adult patient, the most likely diagnosis is a spinal metastasis, perhaps secondary to melanoma.

The differential diagnoses for an intradural extramedullary lesion also include nerve sheath tumours and meningioma. However, a high T1 signal is not characteristic of these lesions.

To take this further, I would like to know if there is a history of malignancy and review any relevant previous imaging. In the absence of a known primary cancer, contrast-enhanced MR imaging of the whole spine and brain and a staging CT scan of the chest, abdomen and pelvis should be arranged to look for a primary malignancy or a phakomatosis such as neurofibromatosis.

Discussion

Intradural extramedullary masses are positioned outside of the spinal cord but within the dural sac. These lesions will neither expand the cord nor indent the thecal sac but will lie within the CSF. These characteristics are easier to see in large, well-defined lesions.

Nerve sheath tumours are associated with the diagnosis of neurofibromatosis in the minority of patients – neurofibromas with NF-1 and schwannomas with NF-2. Neurofibromatosis is an important multisystem disorder in the context of the exams. If you suspect this condition, knowledge of the defined diagnostic criteria and other associated manifestations should be used to formulate your management plan for further imaging.

It may not be possible to distinguish reliably between a neurofibroma and schwannoma as they share similar imaging characteristics. Both tumours may have a "dumbbell" shape. This appearance occurs when the tumour has both an extradural and an intradural component and is narrowed in the middle as it passes through the neural foramen. Over time, the tumour will widen the neural foramen. These features will allow you to distinguish a nerve sheath tumour from metastases and meningiomas.

Metastases in the intradural extramedullary space are relatively uncommon. "Drop" metastases, due to seeding from a primary CNS tumour, are more common in paediatric patients. Metastases from a non-CNS primary tumour are more common in adults and include primary cancers such as melanoma, lung and breast.

This case tests your ability to combine two diagnostic lists – one for the intradural extramedullary mass and the other for a lesion with high T1 signal. This situation is relatively common in the viva setting and tests your ability to process information sensibly when confronted with a number of imaging features. In this case, enhancement is a usual feature of a nerve sheath tumour and a meningioma but the high T1 signal is not. Haemorrhage and fat (lipoma/dermoid) can have a high T1 signal but neither enhance. Melanin produces a high T1 signal and melanoma metastases can enhance, therefore a melanoma metastasis is a sensible proposition in this case.

Pearls

- If the lesion is outside the spinal cord, look at the thecal sac. If it is indented by the lesion from outside, the lesion is extradural. If the lesion lies within the thecal sac and within the CSF, it is intradural extramedullary.
- Substances with a high signal on T1-weighted imaging include subacute haemorrhage (methaemoglobin), fat, protein, melanin and contrast.
- Mention that you would perform contrast-enhanced MRI of the brain and whole spine to look for further lesions and stigmata of phakomatoses such as NF-1.

44.
Extradural spinal mass

"DAMN"

	Condition	Associated features
D	Disc	Commonly multiple associated areas of degenerative disc disease
A	Abscess	Long segment lobulated extradural collection Peripheral enhancement Usually secondary to a primary disc or vertebral infection
M	Metastasis Myeloma	Associated vertebral marrow infiltration contiguous with the mass Commonly multiple
N	Neurofibroma	Indents the theca laterally at the level of exit foramina May have a "dumbbell" appearance

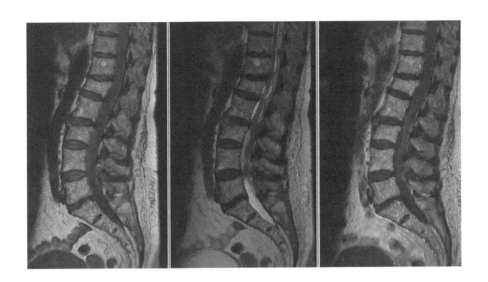

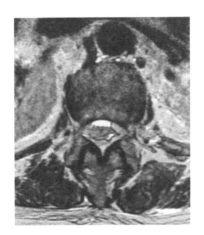

Diagnosis: Extradural abscess

MODEL ANSWER

These are selected T2 and T1 pre- and post-contrast sagittal images of the thoracolumbar spine, with a single axial T2-weighted image.

There is extensive, intermediate T1 and T2 signal material within the spinal canal. This surrounds the cauda equina at the level of L3 and L4, and extends superiorly in the posterior aspect of the spinal canal to at least the T10 level and beyond the upper limit of the provided images. Superiorly, the abnormality has a well-defined wavy contour. CSF can be seen between the abnormality and the spinal cord. On the axial image, the lesion is positioned outside the thecal sac, in keeping with an extradural location. On the post-contrast image, the lesion demonstrates peripheral rim enhancement.

The bone marrow signal is normal and there is no disc abnormality.

In summary, there is an extensive extradural collection in the thoracolumbar spine with peripheral rim enhancement. The findings are in keeping with an extradural abscess. I cannot see a source for the infection on these images.

A spinal extradural abscess is a surgical emergency. I would urgently inform the on-call spinal surgical team of my findings. I would like to see further MR images of the whole spine, as the full extent of the extradural abscess and the source of infection have not been demonstrated.

Discussion

Intraspinal masses may be extradural (as in this case), intradural extramedullary (Case 43) or intramedullary (Case 42). It is vital to localise accurately a spinal mass to one of these three compartments early in your description of a case, as this will lead you to the correct list of differential diagnoses.

In daily practice, there are several conditions that require urgent action when diagnosed. Good examples of these include a tension pneumothorax, leaking abdominal aortic aneurysm, suspected non-accidental injury and spinal cord compression. In the viva, the examiner will want to see that not only can you diagnose these conditions quickly and confidently but also that you recognise the urgency of the situation. A spinal epidural abscess is a surgical emergency due to the risk of spinal cord compression and subsequent paraplegia. The appearances are characteristic and can be differentiated from the other diagnoses described in the table. By beginning your management plan with the simple phase "this is a surgical emergency" you will effectively convey to the examiner that you are a safe radiologist. Failure to clearly demonstrate this understanding may raise doubts about your ability to practice safely.

An extradural abscess usually occurs as a result of local extension from discitis, vertebral osteomyelitis or via haematogenous spread from other sources. It is important to assess the imaging for the primary source of infection.

Degenerative intervertebral disc disease is common and well described. Plain films may show a loss of intervertebral disc space height, vacuum phenomenon and bony sclerosis of the adjacent vertebral end plates. MRI can characterise the type of degenerative disc disease, its precise location and the effect it may have on the adjacent neural structures. You should understand and use the defined descriptions of disc disease such as bulge, protrusion, extrusion and sequestration.

In the presence of spinal trauma or anticoagulation, an extradural haematoma is an important additional differential diagnosis to consider. These will usually appear as a long segment mass with the usual characteristics of blood on an MR image, which are dependent on the age of the haematoma.

Pearls

- A diffuse multi-level epidural abnormality with peripheral enhancement is suggestive of epidural abscess.
- Epidural abscess is a surgical emergency requiring urgent neurosurgical referral.
- Look for evidence of associated discitis or vertebral osteomyelitis.
- Lung, breast and prostate are the most common tumours to metastasise to the spine.

Section 5

Paediatrics

45.
Diffuse periosteal reaction in a child

"CATNIP"

	Condition	Associated features
C	Caffey's disease	Onset <6 months of age; resolved by 1 year Thick irregular periosteal reaction Cortical thickening Commonly involves mandible, clavicle and ribs Less commonly involves long bones with asymmetrical involvement of diaphysis only Soft tissue swelling
A	juvenile idiopathic Arthritis	Variable features including: • osteopenia • erosions • soft tissue swelling
T	Tumour (leukaemia, metastatic neuroblastoma)	Osteopenia Metaphyseal lucent bands (non-specific)
N	Normal (physiological)	Occurs in those aged 1–6 months old Thin periosteal reaction Bilateral and symmetrical Diaphyseal, no metaphyseal involvement
I	Infection, e.g. congenital syphilis	Metaphyseal dense/lucent bands Metaphyseal erosions Bilateral erosions of proximal medial tibial metaphyses (Wimberger's sign)
P	Prostaglandin therapy	Non-specific features May be similar in appearance to Caffey's disease but history of cardiac abnormality

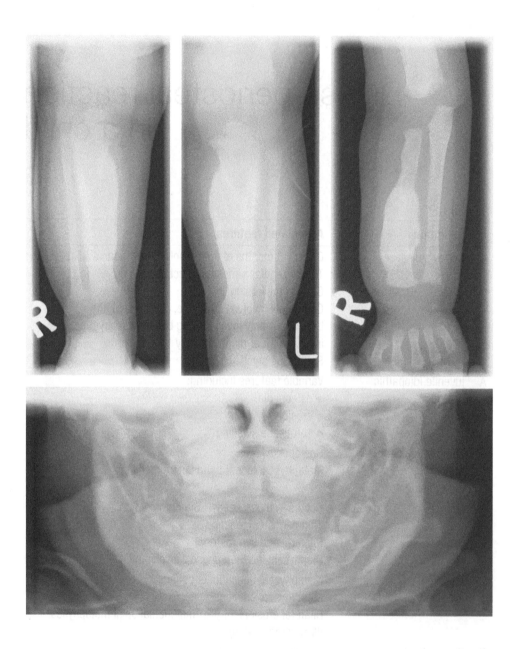

Diagnosis: Infantile cortical hyperostosis (Caffey's disease)

MODEL ANSWER

These are selected plain radiographs of both lower limbs, the right forearm and the mandible of an infant. There is a thick asymmetrical periosteal reaction involving both tibial diaphyses, the right radial diaphysis and the whole mandible. There is no metaphyseal abnormality. The bone density is normal. There is no lucent bone lesion.

In summary, there is marked diffuse periosteal reaction affecting the diaphyses of multiple long bones and the whole mandible. This is most likely due to Caffey's disease. The differential diagnoses include infection, malignancy and prostaglandin therapy.

To take this further, I would review the clinical history and any relevant previous imaging. In particular, I would like to know if there is any history of malignancy and to look for evidence of congenital heart disease on chest radiographs.

Discussion

The periosteum is a thin membrane covering cortical bone. A periosteal reaction is defined as new subperiosteal bone formed in response to soft tissue or osseous disease, detectable by radiographs.

Caffey's disease is a rare self-limiting bone disease of unknown aetiology that affects infants. There is bilateral symmetrical cortical thickening of varying density ranging from subtle periosteal reaction to solid cortical new bone. The mandible is affected in three-quarters of cases. The phalanges are not usually involved. When the long bones are affected, the diaphyses are preferentially involved. The clinical presentation is commonly irritability, fever and localised swelling. Blood tests may reveal a raised ESR and alkaline phosphatase level.

Once you have identified diffuse periosteal reaction, important factors to consider and mention are the bone mineral density, the presence or absence of lucent/lytic lesions and whether there is involvement of the metaphyses. This demonstrates knowledge of the other differential diagnoses – namely, malignancy, inflammatory arthropathy and infection.

Pearls

- Extensive, thick, asymmetrical periosteal reaction with mandibular involvement suggests Caffey's disease.
- Diffuse periosteal reaction with bilateral proximal tibial metaphyseal erosions is typical for congenital syphilis (an "Aunt Minnie").
- Also comment on bone mineral density, the presence of bone lesions and the state of the metaphyses.
- Other important causes of periosteal reaction in children, such as trauma, non-accidental injury and osteomyelitis, are usually focal rather than diffuse.

"MELT"

	Condition	Associated features
M	Metastases Myeloma	Abnormal marrow signal within affected vertebra Associated soft tissue mass May affect multiple vertebrae and involve posterior elements Evidence of primary malignancy elsewhere Less common in the young
E	Eosinophilic granuloma	Uniform flattening of vertebra – "coin-on-edge" or "pancake" vertebra No involvement of posterior elements Preservation of disc space Most often a single vertebra affected Other skeletal features: • lytic skull lesions with a double contour/bevelled edge • long bone lesions, often ill-defined, lytic, diaphyseal
L	Leukaemia Lymphoma	Similar features to metastases and myeloma Usually multiple vertebrae involved Underlying osteopenia in leukaemia
T	TB	Vertebral body destruction, often not uniform May involve disc space (loss of disc height, endplate irregularity), usually at a later stage Abnormal bone marrow signal Epidural, subligamentous and paraspinal abscesses with thick enhancing rims Often affects multiple vertebrae Thoracolumbar kyphosis (gibbus deformity) Most often thoracolumbar spine

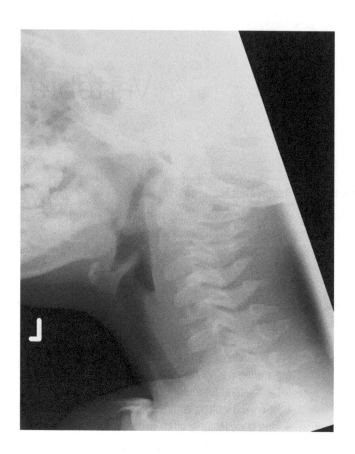

Diagnosis: Eosinophilic granuloma

Definition: A single vertebral body with marked uniform compression but with preservation of the intervertebral disc space

---

MODEL ANSWER

This is a lateral plain film of the cervical spine of a child. There is loss of vertebral body height at C5. The posterior elements appear intact. The sagittal alignment of the C-spine is normal, with no significant prevertebral soft tissue swelling. If there is a history of trauma, I would like to review the remaining films in the standard C-spine trauma series [an AP and odontoid peg view]. In the absence of a trauma history, the most likely diagnosis would be a vertebra plana due to eosinophilic granuloma. However, I would recommend further investigation with MRI, as the differential diagnoses include malignancy and infection.

(MRI sequences are now presented.)

These are selected sagittal T2-weighted images of the cervical spine of the same child. There is a marked and uniform loss of height of the C5 vertebral body, which has a normal bone marrow signal and no evidence of significant oedema. There is mild indentation of the thecal sac by the collapsed vertebral body but no cord compression or evidence of significant associated soft tissue abnormality. The intervertebral disc heights are preserved. No further vertebral lesion is demonstrated.

In summary, the findings are of a C5 vertebra plana. The most likely diagnosis is eosinophilic granuloma. Mycobacterial infection and malignancy should be considered, however, no features of these are demonstrated on these selected images.

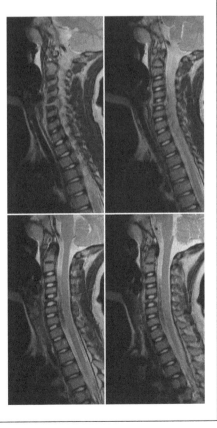

Discussion

Eosinophilic granuloma is the least aggressive form of Langerhans' cell histiocytosis, involving the skeletal and pulmonary systems. It typically affects children of school age (commonest in 4–7 year olds), and is extremely rare in those aged over 20 years. Symptoms include bone pain and swelling. Single lesions are most commonly seen, but multiple lesions can occur. While it has a very varied appearance, some useful points are listed below.

- In the spine, vertebra plana is characteristic.
- In long bones, diaphyseal involvement is common and epiphyseal lesions are very rare.
- The lytic lesions in the pelvis, ribs and long bones may be well or ill-defined, with or without variable periosteal reaction and sclerosis. If aggressive in appearance, they can mimic osteomyelitis and Ewing's sarcoma.
- In the skull, lesions are usually well defined (or "punched out"). Differential involvement of the outer and inner skull tables results in a bevelled edge appearance with a double contour.
- In the mandible and maxilla, destruction of the tooth-bearing alveolar bone can generate a typical "floating teeth" appearance.

Pearls

- Eosinophilic granuloma is the most common cause of a single vertebra plana in a child. However, your differential diagnoses list should include TB and malignancy.
- Also consider neuroblastoma and sarcoma metastases in a child.
- In an adult, metastases and infection are the two most common causes of vertebra plana.
- If presented with a plain film only, recommend or ask to see MR imaging to further assess the bone marrow signal, disc spaces, spinal canal and adjacent soft tissues, to help narrow the list of differential diagnoses.
- A large, associated, epidural/paraspinal abscess with enhancing rims suggests TB.

47.

Multiple wormian bones

"PINT, DOC?"

	Condition	Associated features
P	Pyknodysostosis	Wide skull sutures/fontanelles with delayed closure Small mandible Absent sinuses Absent/hypoplastic clavicles Osteosclerosis of skull base and elsewhere
I	Idiopathic	
N	Normal variant	
T	Hypothyroidism (congenital)	Delayed closure of the fontanelles Small epiphyses with delayed closure
D	Down's syndrome	Hypoplasia of the facial bones and sinuses Atlanto-axial subluxation 11 pairs of ribs Clinodactyly (radial curvature of the little finger)
O	Osteogenesis imperfecta	Osteopenia Deformed and gracile long bones Multiple fractures
C	Cleidocranial dysostosis	Wide skull sutures/fontanelles with delayed closure Normal mandible Normal bone density Absent/hypoplastic clavicles Coxa vara/deformed femoral necks Wide pubic symphysis

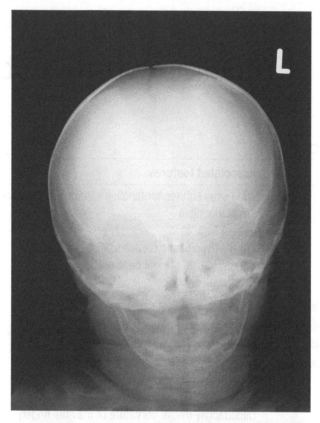

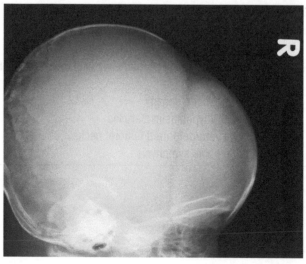

Diagnosis: Idiopathic

Definition: Multiple small bones within the sutures of the skull vault, most commonly the lambdoid suture

---

MODEL ANSWER

These are AP and lateral radiographs of the skull of an infant. The anterior fontanelle has not closed. There are multiple small intrasutural bones within the lambdoid suture. The remainder of the skull is unremarkable. The sutures are not widened. The bone density is normal. The mandible appears normal. No skull fracture. The limited views of the upper thorax on the AP view demonstrate normal clavicles.

In summary, there are multiple wormian bones within the lambdoid suture. There are no secondary features to suggest a specific underlying aetiology. Therefore, this may be idiopathic. Other causes for multiple wormian bones include cleidocranial dysostosis, osteogenesis imperfecta, Down's syndrome, congenital hypothyroidism and pyknodysostosis.

To take this further, I would review the patient history and any relevant previous imaging – in particular, a chest radiograph, to examine the number of ribs and bone density.

Discussion

There are a large number of possible causes for multiple wormian bones. While there may be no features on a skull radiograph that allow you to differentiate between the possible causes, it is worth remembering the more distant secondary features and demonstrating this knowledge. You may be presented with a second related film to allow you to clinch the diagnosis (e.g. a CXR, so that you can count some ribs).

Pearls

- Multiple wormian bones may be idiopathic.
- Look for widened sutures as a sign of an abnormal bone development disorder.
- Assess bone density – there may be osteopenia in osteogenesis imperfecta and osteosclerosis in pyknodysostosis.
- Look at the cervical spine and upper thorax (if included) for any additional abnormalities.
- Distinguish between cleidocranial dysostosis and pyknodysostosis by assessing the bone density and mandible.

48

Posterior fossa mass in a child

	Condition	Associated features
G	Glioma (of brainstem)	Diffuse enlargement of the pons Anterior to the fourth ventricle Often no enhancement
A	Astrocytoma (pilocytic)	Cerebellar lesion Well-defined cyst with a solid enhancing peripheral nodule Large lesions displace the fourth ventricle Hydrocephalus
M	Medulloblastoma	Homogeneous well-defined round mass Hyperdense on pre-contrast CT Uniform enhancement Central – vermis of the cerebellum (80%) Compresses the fourth ventricle "Drop" metastases
E	Ependymoma	Centred on the floor of the fourth ventricle Expands the fourth ventricle Extends through CSF foramina – "toothpaste" tumour Heterogeneous – calcification and cystic change

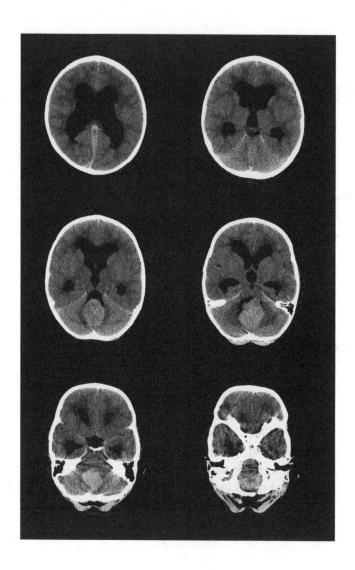

Diagnosis: Medulloblastoma

Definition: An infratentorial space-occupying lesion in a child

---

MODEL ANSWER

These are selected unenhanced axial CT images of the brain of a child. There is a rounded, hyperdense, homogeneous mass in the midline of the posterior fossa. It is centred on the vermis of the cerebellum. The mass extends into the fourth ventricle, which it compresses and displaces to the right. There is associated dilatation of the lateral and third ventricles in keeping with obstructive hydrocephalus. There is no evidence of an associated cystic component, calcification or extension into the basal cisterns.

In summary, there is a homogeneous hyperdense mass within the cerebellar vermis. This compresses the fourth ventricle and causes obstructive hydrocephalus. This is most likely to represent a medulloblastoma. An ependymoma is unlikely as this lesion does not expand of the fourth ventricle. A pilocytic astrocytoma is also unlikely as the mass shows no cystic features.

This is a neurosurgical emergency. I would inform the local neurosurgical unit with a view to urgent treatment of the obstructive hydrocephalus. I would arrange an urgent contrast-enhanced MRI scan of the brain and whole spine to further characterise the lesion and to identify any "drop" metastases within the spine.

Discussion

Whereas the most common cause of a posterior fossa mass in the adult is metastatic disease (most commonly from breast or lung carcinoma), in a child the most common cause is a primary malignancy. These primary tumours have characteristic features, as described in the table. However, there can be a degree of overlap in the imaging features that often prevents a confident diagnosis, especially on CT.

Medulloblastoma is the most common paediatric posterior fossa tumour. It is characterised by rapid growth and high cellularity, which accounts for the hyperdensity on CT and restricted diffusion on MRI. Typically, it arises from the cerebellar vermis or roof of the fourth ventricle, enhances avidly and homogeneously, and causing compression of the fourth ventricle. In contrast, ependymomas are characterised by expansion of the fourth ventricle and can extend through the foramina of Magendie and Luschka. Ependymomas contain areas of focal calcification and cystic change, and therefore have a heterogeneous appearance.

Both medulloblastomas and ependymomas are associated with intradural extramedullary, spinal "drop" metastases. Therefore, it is essential to mention contrast-enhanced MRI of the whole spine when discussing the further management of these paediatric posterior fossa tumours.

Pearls

- Consider the following factors when characterising a posterior fossa mass. Is it central or lateral, hyperdense or cystic, homogeneous or heterogeneous? Can the fourth ventricle be seen – is it compressed, filled or expanded? Does it extend into the basal cisterns? Is there calcification?
- The most common paediatric posterior fossa mass is a medulloblastoma.
- A midline homogeneous and hyperdense mass indicates medulloblastoma.
- A cystic lesion with a small enhancing nodule indicates juvenile pilocytic astrocytoma.
- A heterogeneous lesion expanding the fourth ventricle indicates ependymoma.
- Comment on the presence or absence of hydrocephalus. Obstructive hydrocephalus is a neurosurgical emergency.
- State that you would perform a contrast-enhanced MRI scan of the brain and whole spine to look for "drop" metastases.

49.
Large abdominal mass in a child

"Happy Couples Never Work Over Long Holidays"

	Condition	Associated features
H	Hydronephrosis	Dilated renal pelvis and calyces If due to pelviureteric junction (PUJ) obstruction: normal calibre ureters Most commonly left-sided
C	Cystic kidney disease	Multilocular cystic nephroma: • multiloculated well-defined cystic mass arising from a pole of a kidney, usually lower pole • thick fibrous capsule • enhancing septations • no solid components • claw of distorted renal parenchyma • calcification is rare • does not metastasise – benign mass Multicystic dysplastic kidney: • multiple renal cysts of varying sizes • most commonly unilateral and asymptomatic • fatal if bilateral • no renal parenchyma visible • non-functioning kidney on nuclear MAG3 renogram
N	Neuroblastoma	More common at ages <2 years Large suprarenal/retroperitoneal mass Frequently crosses the midline Calcification typical Encasement of vessels, e.g. aorta, inferior vena cava (IVC), superior mesenteric artery Elevates the aorta anteriorly away from the vertebrae Displaces the kidneys May invade the spinal canal via the neural foramen

	Condition	Associated features
W	Wilms' tumour	More common at ages 2–4 years
		Well-defined, usually solid but sometimes cystic, renal tumour
		"Claw" sign (concavity of renal contour, distorted by tumour)
		Calcification may occur but not as often as in neuroblastoma
		Displacement of vessels
		Sometimes crosses midline
		May invade the renal vein and IVC
O	Ovarian cyst	
L	Lymphoma	Variable appearances:
		• ileocaecal mass with bowel wall thickening
		• mesenteric and retroperitoneal nodal masses
H	Hepatoblastoma	Age <5 years
		Right upper quadrant mass
		Soft tissue mass arising from the right lobe of the liver
		Often heterogeneous with necrosis/haemorrhage/calcifications
		Metastases to lung

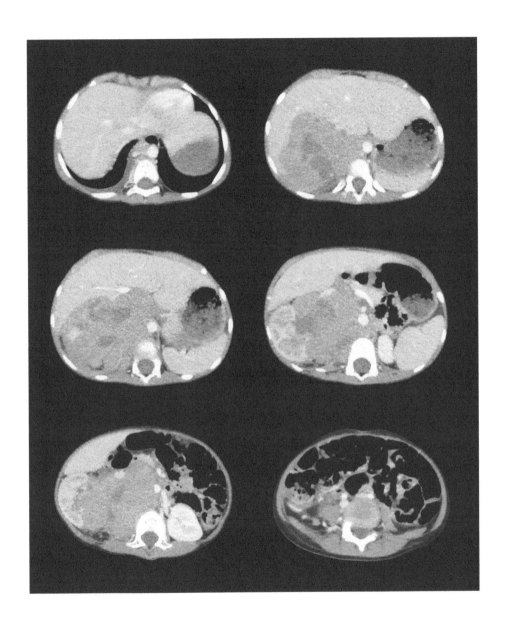

Diagnosis: Neuroblastoma

MODEL ANSWER

These are selected axial post-contrast CT images of a child's abdomen. There is a large, heterogeneous, ill-defined, right-sided retroperitoneal mass. The lesion is centred on the right suprarenal region, displacing the right kidney and right lobe of the liver. The mass crosses the midline and encases the aorta, elevating it anteriorly away from the vertebrae. There are no discernable calcifications. No liver metastases can be seen and there is no obvious involvement of the spinal canal.

In summary, there is a large, retroperitoneal, soft tissue mass, centred on the right suprarenal region, encasing the aorta and displacing the right kidney. This is most likely to represent a neuroblastoma. The differential diagnoses include a Wilms' tumour and lymphoma.

To take this further, I would arrange for the patient to be discussed in the next paediatric multidisciplinary meeting. An MIBG [metaiodobenzylguanidine] scintigraphy scan should be requested to confirm the diagnosis of a neuroblastoma. If there is concern that the lesion is infiltrating the spinal canal, clinically or on imaging, an MRI scan should be requested. A bone marrow aspiration is indicated for accurate staging of bony metastatic disease prior to treatment.

Discussion

There are many causes of an abdominal mass in the paediatric age group. In infants, multicystic dysplastic kidney and hydronephrosis are more commonly seen than tumours. Causes of the latter include PUJ obstruction, primary megaureter, vesicoureteric reflux and posterior urethral valves.

Neuroblastoma and Wilms' tumours are classic cases found in all aspects of the examination. It is very important to know their typical features and how they may be distinguished. In this case, the suprarenal location, encasement of the vessels and displacement of the kidney suggests neuroblastoma. The absence of calcification is atypical. Neuroblastomas also commonly cross the midline. In atypical cases, it may be difficult to tell these two pathologies apart, so both should be included in your list of differential diagnoses when there is a large, solid, perirenal/retroperitoneal mass in a young child.

Neuroblastoma is the most common malignancy in infants. It is a neuroendocrine tumour arising from sympathetic tissue. The most common location is the adrenal gland, followed by elsewhere in the retroperitoneum (sympathetic chain) and the posterior mediastinum. Extensive local spread may be seen, with encasement of vessels and invasion of the spinal canal via the neural foramina. Lymph node, bone, liver and soft tissue metastases are relatively common.

If you are doing well in a viva case of neuroblastoma, you may be asked about the staging system. In Stage 1 and 2 disease, there is localised disease that does not cross the midline. In Stage 3 disease, the tumour involves the midline, and/or there is contralateral nodal involvement. In Stage 4 disease, there is distant metastatic spread. Stage 4S is a special category seen in children under 18 months old, where there is a localised primary tumour and skin, liver or mild bone marrow involvement. This stage has a relatively good prognosis with the potential for spontaneous regression.

A Wilms' tumour is a large, well-defined, heterogeneous renal mass. Several imaging features classically differentiate a Wilms' tumour from a neuroblastoma. A Wilms' tumour will displace rather than encase vessels, is less commonly calcified (10% of cases) and less frequently crosses the midline. A Wilms' tumour may also invade the renal vein with tumour thrombus (10%) that can extend into the IVC. It is also associated with Beckwith–Wiedemann's syndrome and hemihypertrophy.

Pearls

- In neonates, abdominal masses are frequently related to the genitourinary tract, especially hydronephrosis and multicystic dysplastic kidney.
- When presented with a solid, large, retroperitoneal mass in a child, Wilms' tumour, neuroblastoma and lymphoma should be at the top of your list of differential diagnoses.
- An ill-defined retroperitoneal mass with calcification, displacement of the kidney and vascular encasement is likely to be a neuroblastoma.

- When presented with a suspected neuroblastoma, look on the available images for nodal, hepatic, bony and soft tissue metastases as well as for involvement of the spinal canal.
- For further management of neuroblastoma, recommend MDT discussion, bone marrow aspiration, MIBG scintigraphy for accurate staging and an MRI scan of the spine if the tumour lies close to the spinal canal.

50

Neonatal low bowel obstruction

"HAM"

	Condition	Associated features
H	Hirschsprung's disease	Presents within the first 6 weeks of life in term infants Aganglionic bowel is of normal calibre A transition point may be seen and is typically conical Variable proximal dilatation of large bowel
A	Atresia (of ileum, colonic, anal)	Ileal atresia: ● microcolon ● air-fluid levels in dilated small bowel ● no contrast reflux into dilated small bowel at contrast enema Colonic atresia: disproportionately enlarged colon distal to a competent ileocaecal valve Anal atresia: ● clinically apparent ● sacral agenesis ● associated with VACTERL abnormalities (i.e. vertebral anomalies, anal atresia, cardiovascular anomalies, tracheoesophageal fistula, renal and/or radial anomalies, limb defects)
M	Meconium ileus Meconium plug syndrome	Meconium ileus: ● microcolon ● "soap-bubble" lucencies in the terminal ileum (meconium) ● air-fluid levels are rare ● reflux of contrast past distal ileum into dilated small bowel Meconium plug syndrome: ● no microcolon ● variable large bowel dilation ● left colon may be smaller than the right ● plugs of meconium often around splenic flexure

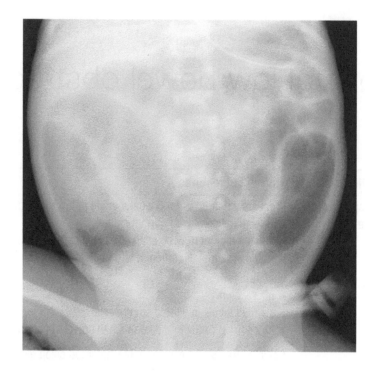

Diagnosis: Meconium ileus

Definition: Neonatal bowel obstruction is considered "low" when the cause is found in the ileum or more distally. It typically presents with delayed passage of meconium and abdominal distension.

MODEL ANSWER

This is an abdominal radiograph of a child. The umbilical clips and absent femoral head ossification centres indicate that this is a neonate. There is a nasogastric tube, the tip of which lies within the stomach.

There are multiple dilated loops of bowel seen throughout the abdomen. There is no evidence of pneumoperitoneum, peritoneal calcifications or portal venous gas to suggest perforation or bowel necrosis.

In summary, the findings are of a low bowel obstruction in a neonate. The likely causes include meconium ileus, meconium plug syndrome, bowel atresia and Hirschsprung's disease.

After discussion with the paediatric surgeons, a contrast enema examination could be performed to assess the cause.

(The contrast enema is then shown.)

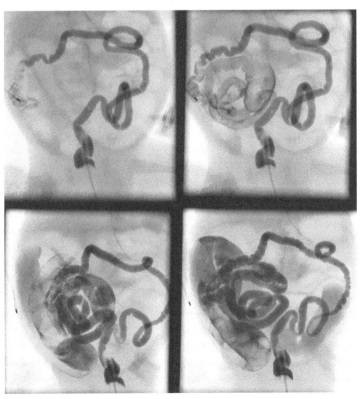

These are selected images from a single contrast enema examination. The whole colon is of small calibre. There are multiple, small, filling defects in the right colon and terminal ileum outlined by contrast.

On the later images, there is reflux of contrast into dilated small bowel. The findings are of meconium ileus. This has a strong association with the diagnosis of cystic fibrosis. I would inform the referring clinician.

Discussion

The presence of multiple loops of dilated bowel in a neonate indicates a low bowel obstruction. It is difficult to differentiate between dilated small and large bowel on AXR in this age group.

Meconium ileus is a very common case seen in both the viva and long case part of the examination. Almost all patients who present with meconium ileus have cystic fibrosis. It is characterised by bowel obstruction secondary to impacted thick meconium at the terminal ileum. On plain radiography, there may be a "soap-bubble" appearance in the right lower abdomen. A contrast enema is essential for diagnosis, showing the typical microcolon and filling defects in the terminal ileum, followed by reflux of contrast into dilated small bowel proximal to the obstruction. The contrast enema is not only diagnostic but also therapeutic. However, repeat enemas may be required to relieve the obstruction. In comparison, there will be no reflux of contrast into the dilated small bowel in ileal atresia.

Meconium plug syndrome is a functional obstruction of the colon. In contrast to meconium ileus, there is no microcolon. The right colon is usually larger than the left, with meconium commonly causing obstruction at the splenic flexure. Hirschsprung's disease can have similar appearances. Contrast enema is again both diagnostic and therapeutic.

In Hirschsprung's disease, there is an aganglionic segment of colon that is unable to relax. This causes a functional colonic obstruction and presents as a failure to pass meconium within the first 48 hours of life. At contrast enema, the aganglionic segment of colon is of normal calibre and the more proximal bowel is dilated. The transition point is classically conical.

Pearls

- If the radiograph is of a neonate (4 weeks old or younger), state this. Look for an umbilical cord clip and absent humeral or femoral head ossification centres.
- If you suspect neonatal low bowel obstruction but are only shown a plain AXR, it is essential to ask for a contrast enema in your management plan.
- Always comment on the presence and position of all catheters and tubes (umbilical artery and/or vein, nasogastric, etc.).
- Comment on the presence and absence of pneumoperitoneum and portal venous gas.
- Is there a microcolon? If yes, then meconium ileus and distal small bowel atresia are the differential diagnoses.
- Meconium ileus is usually associated with underlying cystic fibrosis.

Index

CPD with Radcliffe

You can now use a selection of our books to achieve CPD (Continuing Professional Development) points through directed reading.

We provide a free online form and downloadable certificate for your appraisal portfolio. Look for the CPD logo and register with us at: www.radcliffehealth.com/cpd

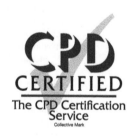

CPD CERTIFIED
The CPD Certification
Service
Collective Mark

T - #0649 - 101024 - C0 - 246/174/14 - PB - 9781908911957 - Gloss Lamination